Asperger Syndrome

A Mindful Approach for Helping Your Child Succeed

(Get a More Extensive Learning About Asperger's and How to Manage It)

Robert Williams

Published By **Bengion Cosalas**

Robert Williams

Asperger Syndrome: A Mindful Approach for Helping Your Child Succeed (Get a More Extensive Learning About Asperger's and How to Manage It)

ISBN   978-1-998927-35-7

No part of this guidebook shall be reproduced in any form without permission in writing from the publisher except in the case of brief quotations embodied in critical articles or reviews.

Legal & Disclaimer

The information contained in this book is not designed to replace or take the place of any form of medicine or professional medical advice. The information in this book has been provided for educational & entertainment purposes only.

The information contained in this book has been compiled from sources deemed reliable, and it is accurate to the best of the Author's knowledge; however, the Author cannot guarantee its accuracy and validity and cannot be held liable for any errors or omissions. Changes are periodically made to this book. You must consult your doctor or get professional medical advice before using any of the suggested remedies, techniques, or information in this book.

Upon using the information contained in this book, you agree to hold harmless the Author from and against any damages, costs, and expenses, including any legal fees potentially resulting from the application of any of the information provided by this guide. This disclaimer applies to any damages or injury caused by the use and application, whether directly or indirectly, of any advice or information presented, whether for breach of contract, tort, negligence, personal injury, criminal intent, or under any other cause of action.

You agree to accept all risks of using the information presented inside this book. You need to consult a professional medical practitioner in order to ensure you are both able and healthy enough to participate in this program.

Table Of Contents

Chapter 1: Asperger's Syndrome and Adolescents

The teenage years are a time of existence that takes vicinity among childhood and adulthood. Adolescence is a period of physical, mental, and social transformation.

Puberty, or the method of sexual adulthood, is one of the physical changes. Adolescence is a time of large famous bodily change in pinnacle, weight, and appears, in phrases of sexual development. This generation of speedy improvement is due to the inner release of hormones.

Hormones are defined as "a chemical, often a peptide or steroid, synthesized thru manner of 1 tissue and transported with the useful aid of the circulate to every other to effect physiological function, together with growth or metabolism."

Hormones in excessive concentrations create fast physiological trade, that could make a young person sense disturbing and uncertain. The speedy physical modifications also can create ache and identity uncertainty, specifically in younger human beings with AS who take consolation in predictability and sameness.

Adolescent highbrow modifications encompass both cognitive and emotional improvement. The most crucial difference in teens is their growing functionality to cope with and clear up stressful conditions of developing complexity.

This functionality to clear up troubles at extra modern ranges can be obscured at times through way of the emotional overload professional inside the course of this era of transition, however it is present and will become extra obvious as soon due to the fact the teen has adjusted to his or her bodily and highbrow changes.

The social versions at some point of children are closely tied to the sexual and physical modifications that rise up. Teenagers have become extra concerned in social interactions and being familiar socially.

Adolescents are much more likely to pick out out out pals and pals above mother and father or guardians. This is actual for the extremely good majority of teens, even people with Asperger's Syndrome.

Such is applicable for children who do no longer have pals but want to, similarly to folks that pick out no longer to have buddies. This is a length of developing cognizance in peer social conduct.

It can be determined out through way of an prolonged interest in teen clothing, makeup, hair styles, tune, teenager- or younger-individual hobbies, interacting with others on the internet, and noticing the possibility sex, in preference to via an better large form of social connections, as it's miles with younger people who do not have troubles. During teenhood, social adjustments consist of the preference for a terrific identity in addition to a deeper records of oneself.

Teenage years even as a person's increase drives or, in a few conditions, eases him or her in the route of a more longing for independence in everyday lifestyles. This length seems to force the bulk of teens to be extra sociable than at each one of a kind difficulty in their life.

This is an top notch time to work on building social competency, but in depth concentration on this location can be extra beneficial if dealt with inside the person with AS's later adolescent years.

Because teenhood is this type of turbulent and complex time for everybody, the actual freedom to find out social interactions can be superb treated as soon as the bodily, emotional, and mental adjustments were described and the frame structure has reduced.

Chapter 2: Asperger Syndrome Diagnosis

Asperger Syndrome is more tough to diagnose than exclusive ASDs. This is specifically proper for teens, who certainly might in all likelihood seem to undergo a normal adolescent section. The key to supporting a person with Asperger Syndrome is to become aware about the problem early and broaden a program or remedy for that person.

However, which will do so, one want to be looking for symptoms and signs and installation whether or not or not they are because of Asperger's or some other infection, in conjunction with ADHD. Moreover, a few clinical medical doctors make the mistake of misdiagnosing a affected person with a one-of-a-type kind of autism, first-rate to later find out that the affected individual's state of affairs is on account of Asperger's.

Individuals who're suspected of getting Asperger Syndrome can be closely monitored for indicators or symptoms a high-quality manner to confirm whether or not or now not or now not they've got the contamination or now not.

An superb technique to accomplish that is to have a observe the character's social interactions and decide whether or not or no longer some thing is awry. Because ladies and men with Asperger Syndrome regularly have a speciality or a particular ability, it's also crucial to check for uncommon competencies or interests that may make contributions to a possible affected man or woman's social pain.

Is Asperger's Syndrome inherited?

The autism spectrum disease has deep genetic underpinnings. When all autism signs and symptoms and signs and signs, from mild to excessive, are included, the matching possibility for equal twins is ninety%. A 1/three of the dad and mom of a infant with Asperger's syndrome will revel in at the least some of the signs and symptoms indexed above.

When a decide sees his very very very own symptoms in his youngster or a lady recognizes them in her associate, the illness is frequently identified most effective in maturity. Despite this genetic foundation, there can be no evidence of a selected organic etiology in the imply time. In particular families, absolutely one of a kind gene combos may be implicated, and there may be a couple of underlying mind ailment or abnormality.

According to at least one time-commemorated idea, people with Asperger's syndrome and one-of-a-type autistic illnesses lack a "concept of mind" – the intuitive cognizance that others have mind and feelings. As a give up end result, they are now not able to picture themselves into the mind of others as a way to anticipate their answers. Instead, they should laboriously deduce certainly one of a kind people's sentiments, intentions, and interests using specific rules.

That's meant to present an reason for why a person who can recognize intricate technological approaches could not hold a everyday communique. Brain scans exhibit that once we interpret facial expressions, the amygdala, a hub of emotion, is lively in the majority human beings. The prefrontal cortex, a middle of judgment and planning, lighting fixtures up in people with Asperger's syndrome. They are contemplating about the meaning of the statement as opposed to reacting to it speedy.

Chapter 3: A few of the issues that young adults with Aspergers confront

1. Weird linguistic use

Individuals with AS may have a whole lot of verbal talents starting from no longer on time to superior. Peaks and valleys are terms used to explain the great sort of linguistic abilities. Language capacity peaks and dips can complex to others and are frequently elaborate for the man or woman with AS.

Great expressive vocabulary, accurate speech articulation, and strong sentence employer are common peaks. The lowlands are characterised with the beneficial resource of a lack of know-how and social use of language.

It is natural for listeners to think that a person with a massive, expressive vocabulary and proper grammar may be able to have interaction and join properly with others. This presumption is based on the truth that most increase, which include language skills acquisition, proceeds in an first-rate and ordinary way.

While all of us has strengths and barriers, the peaks and troughs in language improvement placed in young humans and adults with AS are often larger than those seen in the popular public.

This arises because of the truth the splendid talents are extremely good and the lousy competencies are very prone, ensuing in a larger discrepancy than might be discovered in a normal populace. It is the difference that leads listeners to be confused as soon as they'll be looking for to recognize the speaker's thing of view.

2. Pragmatics is the social use of language.

This would be the series of norms that determines how people use language in social situations. Social regulations are regularly unwritten and unsaid, complex, and continuously evolving, and they govern honestly all factors of social interplay.

These encompass, but are not restricted to, speaking in instantaneous touch with others, nonverbal communication, welcomes and farewells, verbal exchange, the speech act, powerful listening, and the roles of speaker and listener as they relate to gender, age, and function. Individuals who do not have AS discover it quite clean to word pragmatic violations, which lead to not unusual misunderstandings.

It is vital to understand that pragmatic breaches get up for a number of motives. The character with a social pragmatic trouble may not maintain near the which means that of maximum of the social requirements of language usage and, as a stop result, may not adhere to the policies as strictly as different people.

He may be able to look at or even enforce a rule, however it does no longer seem natural to him, therefore the rule of thumb is less strictly enforced. It is from time to time essential to in reality consider that this need is essential for first rate relationships.

This is specially right almost approximately greets and farewells. Because he won't want or require others to use hiya and farewells, it might be difficult for him to genuinely comprehend and accept as true with that others do. This isn't uncommon considering the fact that every person see the area and our relationships thru our very own lens, which has been shaped with the beneficial useful resource of our very personal personal reports.

If I don't have any want for welcomes and farewells whilst a person enters or quits a room, I can also moreover discover it tough to realise and take delivery of that that may be a principal requirement for others. It's understandable that I have to not truly take delivery of this preference of others, wondering that requiring precise social conduct is stupid, if not ludicrous.

A person experiencing social pragmatic issues may additionally moreover furthermore have problem with the speech act, which includes sentence production, phrase desire, sound articu-lation, and paralinguistic elements. This conflict may additionally additionally generate anxiety on its personal, however whilst mixed with social interactions with others, it motives massive fear.

This combination of expressive language issues, social hurdles, and tension can result in fantastic pragmatic problem beginning a communicate, keeping a topic of mutual hobby, and adhering to a subject of common interest.

In this example, there are just too many variables to manipulate for the social engagement to be clean and exciting for each the speaker and the listener, and the individual with AS need help from the conversational companion to development past this issue.

Whenever all the speaker and the listener draw close the underlying nature of the social pragmatic stressful conditions, pragmatic disturbing conditions may be decreased. The problems are given now not intentionally misinform the verbal exchange associate or to portray oneself as definitely self-absorbed and narcissistic, however rather due to underlying social pragmatic false impression. This is the vicinity wherein neurotypicals (NTs) have to enhance their comprehension of the person with AS if proper development is to be made.

Someone with standard social pragmatic skills want learn how to suppose in autism through adopting the attitude of the person with social pragmatic problems. Rather than disregarding the speak and shunning the person, NTs ought to make a compromise and make bigger knowledge to the person that is struggling within the mean time.

Acceptance, compromise, and know-how are supportive traits with a purpose to assist teenagers and adults with AS to exercising and use the social abilties needed to decorate social competence.

three. Nonverbal communication

Teenagers and adults with AS usually warfare to recognize nonverbal symptoms from others, in conjunction with eye contact, facial gestures, body postures, and gestures.

Individuals who fail to successfully take a look at nonverbal conversation are vulnerable to persistent disagreements with others, even folks that are familiar with them and the character in their troubles. Nonverbal verbal exchange debts for as a good buy as fifty 5% of the meaning in face-to-face communication, for that reason deficiencies in this vicinity can notably impair social relationships.

4. Changing one's thoughts-set

For the adolescent with AS, the incapacity or inclined factor to peer a situation via the eyes of a few different man or woman can motive large misinterpretation and large social issues. Because records differs, it is hard to mention to what quantity mindset-taking negatively affects social connections of teenagers and adults with AS, despite the fact that maximum agree that attitude-taking is an hassle.

Prominent college students have proposed that a key illness of autism is impaired mind-set-taking. However, this isn't the case with AS. In Hans Asperger's authentic description of his patients, he remarked on his topics' sturdy attitude-taking talents; he is defined in his explanation of the ailment as pronouncing that there was "an capability to engage in a positive shape of introspection and to be a decide of character."

It appears that many, if now not all, teenagers and adults with AS battle with perspective-taking to some extent. While those competencies do not appear to make bigger instinctively, many young adults and adults react favorably to planned education in this place.

5. Compassion

Compassion is one of the maximum normally misunderstood components of AS. Empathy is the capacity to come to be privy to with some other individual's emotions, mind, or attitudes. It is the capability to be sad at the equal time as others are unhappy and afraid whilst others are afraid.

Individuals who do not understand AS often witness someone with AS's conduct and social errors and end that they lack the potential to come to be privy to with the feelings, mind, or attitudes of others, but this is truely no longer actual. People with AS might also have sturdy feelings approximately a big variety of troubles, even those who effect others.

Difficulties usually arise while the person with AS fails to be conscious another person's ache or situation, however while the feeling is determined, empathy follows. Teens and adults may additionally require a bit greater time to device the verbal exchange and add clarity to the message, or they may require extra time to formulate a response.

At instances, they may need to be understood after they react to an emotional circumstance with what appears to be a loss of compassion, because of the truth empathy isn't always an all-or-not whatever hassle.

6. Concentration and agency

Many teenagers and adults with Asperger's syndrome war with paying interest and staying organized. Some people have a restrained interest span, which makes it tough to be aware of some thing for greater than a quick quantity of time. Others struggle with hypervigilant hobby, which compels them to focus on the whole thing. Others are with out troubles distracted with the aid of way of approach of out of doors sensory stimuli, while others are without difficulty distracted thru interior mind.

Attention deficits are sometimes observed with hyperactivity. This may be an problem for others. Many teenagers and adults say that they have been to begin with identified with Attention Deficit Disorder (ADD) or Attention Deficit Hyperactivity Disorder (ADHD) before being identified with AS (ADHD).

This seems to be because of factors: the behaviors are a good deal less tough to phrase, and lots of clinicians are greater experienced and snug with this restoration prognosis. Some humans have AS in addition to ADD or ADHD, although this is not the case for every body.

Issues focusing interest will result in social issues. Attending to a conversation accomplice is essential for effective conversation. When human beings battle to pay interest within the course of a communicate, they may be more likely to break, talk over others, shift the state of affairs, misread the message, or be misunderstood.

Clear communique necessitates that each the speaker and the listener be absolutely concerned inside the communique. Full participation necessitates paying interest past the ideal bodily function to being attentive to and comprehending every word, similarly to studying each verbal exchange companion's motive.

Poor attendance may also moreover reason misconception and sickness in all areas of existence. This reasons issues with keeping appointments, being on time, missing interest interviews, missing final dates, and forgetting birthdays. Being disorga-nized may be a hard experience.

7. Distinctive and deep passions

Most human beings with AS display off enthusiastic situation with specific interests or extreme interest in ordinary subjects or gadgets. Topics which consist of memorizing sports records or having an abnormally intense fixation on a sure trouble, which includes the weather, are examples of particular pastimes.

Many of these issues, which includes sturdy interest in foreigners, birthdates, automobile registration plates, or bus routes, are super. Some people's hobbies variety regularly, however others may additionally stay with a unmarried ardour for decades.

Powerful pastimes provide each blessings and drawbacks. The benefits of having robust unique pursuits encompass the ability to deliver leisure, entertainment and enjoyment time, offer higher regularity in life, permit conversations, permit a person to emerge as an expert in a first-rate assignment, and, frequently, cause a a hit project.

The terrible of specific pastimes is that they can call for a vast amount of time, that could interfere with the time required to investigate one among a kind skills and capacities, collectively with the ones required for developing social interactions and life abilties important for residing independently.

8. Trouble in combining sensory statistics

Numerous teenagers and adults with AS have heightened sensory reactions and battle to adjust sensory statistics. Sound, moderate, touch, texture, flavor, scent, pain, movement, temperature, and special stimuli can all purpose problems. These surprising reactions may also additionally range from mild underreactions to strong overreactions to a sense.

It is idea that the most worried device does not effectively interpret sensory input, resulting in a response this is each lower or better than that decided in those who do now not have AS. With well based totally totally remedy, integration and reactions to sensory records can be advanced.

Many young adults and adults declare that as they grow to be older, their capability to deal with sensory troubles improves. Some claim that this development stems from being capable of cope better in present day. Others declare that as adults, they now have extra have an impact on over their surroundings and might regulate or keep away from unpleasant sports activities. Others, alternatively, report locating pills that alleviate their sensory issues.

Sensory stimulation can motive modest to intense reactions. Of path, the more potent the reaction, the extra probably it's miles that the stimuli may additionally additionally intrude with a person's life. Interference is normally generated while a person restricts his interest to be able to avoid being assaulted through the use of the use of unsightly sensory sensations.

If a person is allergic to particular fragrances, she may be no longer capable of enter new ingesting locations or sections of town, experience on a crowded bus or metro, or be among groups of people who are sporting perfumes or colognes. Because heady scent and taste are so in detail related, her consuming options may be restricted.

Food restraints will absolutely restrict social alternatives and possibilities due to the fact such a lot of cultures socialize round food, which consist of sharing food collectively. Adverse sensory reactions may be unpleasant, tension-inducing, uncomfortable, and draining.

Chapter 4: Developing social abilities

In order to flourish, social competencies must be evolved. Social skills are the competencies that we are required to make use of in our society to interact with others. They are founded on our society's social necessities and educate us what attitudes and moves are deemed normal, suitable, and anticipated in a given social context.

For you and me, social talents are essential due to the truth they allow us to engage with a in addition predictably, permitting us to better apprehend and be understood. Misunderstandings are incredibly difficult to avoid inside the absence of an agreed-upon social way of interacting. It is important that we be able to interact with readability.

It is likewise critical to apprehend that individuals with nicely-advanced social talents are frequently visible as succesful and a success thru manner of others in their tradition. They also are significantly cherished through the usage of others, at the same time as people who fail to apprehend social competencies are often considered as incompetent with the useful resource of society.

Isolation, emotions of loneliness, frustration, rejection, and espresso vanity can end result from a failure to recognize suitable social skills. It is critical for oldsters with AS to recognize that their failure is because of their impairment, not to a scarcity of training or dedication.

Interpersonal talents are critical for society due to the truth they offer order and shape even as additionally transmitting our manner of lifestyles's principles, values, motives, social roles, language, and emblems from one era to the subsequent. All of these trends and behaviors are appeared as essential for survival thru society.

How to Use Social Skills to Improve Your Relationships

1. Associates

Associates are people with whom we have were given a passing dating. These relationships are frequently shaped because of a common experience. Schoolmates, coworkers, bus drivers, provider businesses, instructors, professors, store clerks, friends, waiters, attendants, and parishioners are examples of pals. Associates are large because they constitute the majority of people with whom most parents have common contact. Associates inhabit commonplace areas and beneficial aid with regular existence sports activities. They moreover supply a large organisation of people from which functionality pals is probably determined. The college education of conversation sophistication desired with the aid of this shape of courting varies, however in favored, the ones relationships require easy styles of verbal exchange which includes greetings and farewells, smooth wishes, or first-class climate talk paired with nonverbal gestures which include a grin, nod, wave, or eye gaze. While most pals want sincere communique, greater elements should possibly make acquaintance degree interactions particularly prone to misinterpretation for teenagers and adults with AS.

In many instances, the very splendid way to talk with friends is to growth a script or a list that has all of the information you may need for severa varieties of touch. Jonathan grow to be at the start properly organized for his new journey at the bus. He end up aware that he had to introduce himself to the purpose pressure after which divulge the ideal address of his place of business. Unfortunately, after he set up a pattern, he forgot to supply the important records in case of a trade.

Learning to have interaction with buddies can be as easy as watching those humans on your existence who in shape the classification of acquaintance, considering that person's characteristic in your lifestyles, and getting prepared an good enough script that consists of the essential facts to help you to your interactions with every associate.

The following are the levels to extra green interpersonal contacts with pals:

1. Make a list of the names or titles of individuals in your life who you regard to be

pals. It is useful to keep this statistics in a pocket e book or non-public digital assistant (PDA); consist of classmates, instructors, coworkers, provider vendors, clerks, economic organization tellers, and bus drivers.

2. Alphabetize the listing so that you can without problem discover the records at the same time as you want it.

3. Identify each acquaintance's essential feature.

four. Make a listing of the vital trouble information you'll want to hold with each acquaintance. Make advantage of effective take a look at-taking strategies.

five. Pay interest to the human beings in your list, write down what you phrase, and bear in mind everybody's importance in your lifestyles.

For example, a monetary organization employee will will let you with coins requests, deposits, and transfers. Keep in thoughts that it is important for monetary group employees to be beneficial and offer assist to the bank's customers. A teller may additionally moreover look like exceptional and talkative. You may additionally look at this person starting a welcome with a weather commentary or enquiring approximately your well-being.

This is known as "small communique." Other customers inside the queue in advance of you will be making "small communication" in reaction to the tellers. You may also see the teller saying, "How may additionally furthermore I help you in recent times?" So, on the equal time as making prepared a screenplay for the financial employer teller, you can need to put together factors: one to reply to "small conversation," and the opportunity to make your precise banking need.

6. When making "small chat," it is crucial to apprehend that many people pick out out secure, predictable, and impersonal subjects

at the same time as speaking with buddies, together with short remarks on the present day country of the weather, which include "It is awfully hot these days." Many humans inquire about the alternative character's nicely-being, which consist of "How are you in recent times?"

This may be deceptive because of the fact the most effective asking the query is essentially welcoming the individual in choice to inquiring approximately their real properly-being. Almost always, the acquaintance may additionally react to this sort of question with "I'm OK" or "I'm high-quality."

7. Depending in your findings, create a short script of the social stumble upon on your pocket ebook or PDA that you feel will bring about a nice engagement with every touch. Remember to apply clean, succinct, and courteous language. Include reminders that permits you to remind you to be expressive in your conversation and body language.

8. Use your pocket e book or PDA to rehearse and amazing your scripts. It is right to preview your script before meeting with a associate. For instance, in case you are heading to do grocery purchasing or to the bank, preview your scripts in advance than going.

2. FAMILIES

The name "own family" can observe to a substantial collection of people, however on this ebook, "family" refers to the ones individuals who represent a social institution along with mother and father or guardians, their youngsters, and people who're at once connected to them, consisting of grandparents, uncles, aunts, and cousins.

In present day Western civilization, the circle of relatives is frequently considered as a place in which closeness, love, and accept as true with are promoted and in which humans also can moreover escape the pressures of a difficult worldwide.

Families bring love, safety, assist, warmth, compassion, sympathy, and training. While it also includes assumed that people of families will continuously love, consider, and understand each different, this isn't always the case. Families, like each exclusive enterprise organization, are crafted from humans.

The truth that individuals are engaged approach that there will be issues on occasion. Many of the issues that rise up among individuals of households revolve on communication.

Communication can be hard in any family, however it's miles extra tough in families whilst one or extra people have communication troubles. The unique and pervasive communique problems that teens and adults with AS have may be very anxious for them every person of their circle of relatives.

Excellent communique is the essential component to keeping extraordinary connections amongst circle of relatives individuals. The following are the degrees to stepped forward verbal exchange:

1. Develop a willingness to boom conversation and social contact amongst your self and your circle of relatives. This might be tough for the cause that you could harbor resentment or animosity toward circle of relatives members because of poor relationships within the past. It is tough to move on from previous grievances, however it's far viable.

2. Conduct an sincere assessment of your contribution to previous grievances or verbal exchange challenges. The most difficult trouble of this segment is staying targeted to your very very personal characteristic in the social and conversation challenges. You should keep in thoughts that you can most effective regulate your self; you can't alternate every person else.

three. Using the evaluation, take a look at out your social and conversation talents. As the speaker or listener, you may have a look at that you have failed in a few manner. You can also comprehend that you have not made the vital efforts to maintain exquisite communique with own family individuals, or that if issues have emerged, you have got got failed to apologize or searching for a few form of resolution for the false impression.

If such is the situation, you'll possibly beg the member of the family to forgive you and provide you a fresh begin. True, communique disturbing conditions are an thing of life with AS, consequently they may arise. It is likewise real that maximum people respond favorably to an apology and are normally inclined to offer any individual a second hazard.

four. Choose strategies that will help you decorate your verbal exchange within the regions you have diagnosed as tough. As a public speaker, you may need to:

1. Use smooth, direct language.

2. Be aware of paralinguistic clues that could assist you carry more which means.

three. Use nonverbal signals to aid your announcement.

4. Pay interest to the audience and, if critical, adapt your message.

five. Be conscious of the legal recommendations of discourse.

6. Think on what you have got were given heard.

7. If you are unsure, ask inquiries.

5. Be open and honest in conjunction with your family members. Share your troubles, hopes, and desires. Tell them how they're succesful to help you, after which be willing to simply accept their assist. If you do no longer need assistance in a positive situation, explicit this well.

With household own family, like with everybody else with whom you desire to have an high-quality connection, you may need to utilize global contributors of the family in preference to stark honesty.

Diplomacy is a courteous and complex way of managing others. This permits you to particular your self whilst moreover contemplating the requirements of others.

3. FRIENDS

Friends are two or more human beings who have a reference to each precise that involves mutual love, respect, take delivery of as proper with, and unconditional recognition. When people bear in mind themselves to be pals, it typically approach that they've identified mutual pursuits.

Friends are frequently useful and supportive of every other. They spend time together doing subjects they both experience. They are worried about the protection and happiness of each specific and ask every one-of-a-kind questions. They wait and pay attention closely to the answer after asking a question. They help each unique even though it's a ways tough for them or when they would love to do some thing else.

When a friend makes a mistake or has a viewpoint that varies from their personal, they attempt to recognize. Friends are committed to each other and exercising prioritizing each other's interests over their very own. Friends assist each different, try and understand each other, are dedicated to every extraordinary, and preserve but every other business enterprise.

Friendships do no longer typically include romantic interests, however they might result in more close relationships with romantic interests. If both person realizes that a friendship has superior proper into a sexual appeal, it is vital that each men and women percent the identical choice, otherwise the connection might be damaged.

Nothing is greater complicated than one buddy growing romantic love for a few different and the feelings no longer being again. It is vital to understand that no longer everyone locations the equal fee on having pals. Some people select to loaf around with just one friend, whilst others prefer to hold out with a group of pals.

Some young adults and adults with AS can also moreover select to have no friends as all. In this situation, the youngster's or character's family can be extra worried approximately her having friends than she is ready herself.

It is vital to understand that the advantages of getting pals may be severa for those who preference them. Friends may additionally additionally make lifestyles extra exciting.

Through friendship and entertainment, they will supply pleasure and excitement. They provide recommend and is probably beneficial during annoying instances. People who've friends are notion to be an awful lot less lonely, happier, have better shallowness, and are more a success.

The following are the ranges to developing new buddies.

1. Research the dreams of friendship. Friendships are consensual connections that necessitate cooperation, loyalty, mutual aid, the sharing of commonplace hobbies, spending time collectively, being interested in each exclusive's properly-being, helping every one-of-a-type, being attentive to each different, trying to understand every extraordinary, and setting the pal's pastimes inside the the front of your very very very own.

Make a listing of your private passions. This is large because of the truth friendships are regularly based on shared pastimes.

2. You are genuinely prepared to look for a associate. This person is probably a person you recognize, a person you bypass to school with, someone you discern with, a person you recognize from a membership or church, or a person who lives on your metropolis.

You'll want to discover someone who shares your pursuits or has pastimes which might be just like yours. This will want you looking at, noticing, and attending to important people for your social surroundings. To create friends, you need to be aware about special human beings for an extended enough term to find out whether or not you've got were given some element in not unusual.

three. When you choose a functionality pal based totally on your observations and it appears which you have a shared hobby, strike up a conversation approximately it. It is honestly useful to growth a list of questions earlier to persuade your talk. You may also moreover additionally collect a bulleted list or write a whole screenplay. A listing will assist you hold in thoughts topics and preserve you on direction while talking with a potential pal.

A script will can help you exercise your discussion in advance than speakme with the capacity friend, enhancing your consolation degree with the upcoming chat. You may additionally additionally compose a script that focuses only to your interests, or you could embody a few self-disclosure.

Self-disclosure is even as you tell a person about your impairment as a way to make easy moves or mannerisms that might have previously uncovered your demanding situations. Because of the benefit with which human beings with traditional social competencies be conscious difficulties with pragmatics, many different people have already detected that a social hassle exists. When humans understand the person of the situation, they typically reply in reality.

four. To make sure fulfillment, restriction the quantity of time spent on the initial get-collectively. Developing friendships necessitates focusing your hobby on the opposite character, which may be taxing after a while. During it slow together, make sure you awareness at the recounted prerequisites of friendship.

five. It is OK to call your new capability buddy after a quick time body, probably a week. Remember that you want to be remembered as a devoted buddy, now not a bothersome pal. Tell her you had a pleasing time and desire she did as properly. You may additionally furthermore inquire approximately her thoughts approximately the collection.

If she says it did not circulate nicely or shows that she does no longer need to do it all over again, it's miles wise to invite her how the get-collectively could possibly have long long gone better. Tell her you would need to pay interest her mind on how matters went inside the hopes that topics should pass higher subsequent time or that you may test from the enjoy.

6. Take some time to keep in mind and contemplate in your potential pal's terms. Consider and replicate on your very own observations. Make a listing of any pointers you have for a manner to enhance the state

of affairs or such situations inside the future. You can also moreover speak those thoughts with the possible buddy or with someone you understand properly.

7. If the initial attempt is unsuccessful, resume your look for a pal. Don't be disheartened when you have to undergo those approaches numerous times earlier than you discover a chum. Many people spend their complete lives with excellent one or pals and assume themselves fortunate.

Chapter 5: Advice for Coping with Individuals Who Have Asperger Syndrome

A individual with Asperger Syndrome calls for all the love and manual he can gain from his circle of relatives and buddies. This is in particular essential for a teenager, because it's miles at this age that a person research bodily and emotional modifications that he may not recognise.

If you've got were given a cherished one with Asperger's syndrome, it's far important that you provide him with emotional manual and be specially patient with him. Remember that almost all of his behaviors stem from his false impression of tactics social policies need to take a look at to each person.

Here are some hints to help you manipulate with a cherished one that has Asperger Syndrome:

1. Maintain a everyday time table.

Structure is crucial within the life of a person with Asperger Syndrome. Having to do duties at regular periods in some unspecified time in the future of the day allows to hold him calm and reminds him that the whole thing is splendid. Set a time restriction for his activities—meals, assignments, and amusement—and adhere to it. If you have got were given an Asperger's infant or adolescent, you can moreover installation a nighttime for him.

2. Take it slow. A individual with Asperger Syndrome, particularly a infant, is rarely aware that what he says or does is hurtful to others. Be more affected man or woman with him and take transport of his flaws, together with tactlessness, temper outbursts, and mood swings. Remember to be moderate and compassionate with him, and to conform your expectations for his conduct and different factors.

three. Reproach and punish with love. If you may reprimand a kid or adolescent with Asperger Syndrome, offer an reason behind why and inform him which you despite the fact that love him even in case you want to punish him for some factor. If you are handling an adult with the condition, you could criticize him for his behavior, but acquire this in a being concerned manner, telling him what he did poorly and what he have to do proper in the upcoming destiny.

four. Form a reliable help enterprise. You can't do it on your personal. Dealing with a person who has Asperger Syndrome also can sap your energy in case you do all of it for your private. Get help from a fixed of relied on own family humans, buddies, and coworkers. Allow them to be your sounding board for any issues you will be having along side your Asperger's-affected cherished one.

Allow them that will help you with minor obligations to lessen your load. If you do now not have a help group, you may probably set up counseling or remedy to assist relieve tension occasionally. Remember that a wonderful way to assist the one that you love in dealing with his disorder, your highbrow and emotional fitness must be in well operating order.

5. Prepare a list of verbal and physical clues. Create a device of codes that you and the only which you love also can use to find if considered one of you calls for some thing from the opportunity. Using verbal cues or gestures may also moreover assist you take a break and put off the priority till every of you are in a better mood to deal with it.

6. Recognize pressures in his surroundings. Take the time to discover approximately what reasons panic assaults and a way to prepare for them. These might be troubles at college or at art work, peer stress, or maybe a love situation. Prepare solutions for a manner to deal with them and provide propose on how to overcome them.

7. Simplify your manner of living.

A person with Asperger Syndrome can also moreover have rituals that make him enjoy secure, similarly to favored gadgets and places that offer him with a sense of belonging. Cultivate this emotion by using the use of refusing to result in on him doing some thing else which you agree with is higher for him. Instead, provide him your whole assist for an interest or skills wherein he's devoting his time, so long as his pursuit does not endanger or damage him in any manner.

Be realistic on your expectancies. Do now not anticipate to do the entirety in a short time body. Accept that there can be setbacks alongside the road, and that the objectives you put at the outset of your experience won't be reached without a doubt.

If you're the determine of a child with Asperger Syndrome, it's miles most high-quality in case you and your partner can reach an settlement on a manner to manipulate your toddler's condition. This includes remedy, counseling, and the restrictions you need to set up for your little one. Attend Asperger Syndrome workshops or meetings to have a look at extra about the state of affairs, after which communicate it collectively together with your accomplice or partner.

Discuss the matter openly as a own family and provide you with opportunity solutions. If important, are looking for outdoor assistance, which incorporates by way of using enrolling in couple's counseling.

9. Look for the satisfactory school on your toddler. It is really useful to invest in a private school that caters for your toddler's specific dreams if you can offer you with the cash for to pay the charges. However, in case you receive as real with that a network university is the great alternative, go to the relaxation of your circle of relatives and study the college's shape, ideals, and records of tolerance for people with ASD.

10. Discuss the scenario with the character in query. Your loved one need to recognize what goes on with him and why he appears to be particular from exceptional humans his age. This is particularly essential for teens with

Asperger Syndrome, who face the most try to comply in.

To help the one that you love get keep of himself and alter to his surroundings, he should first apprehend his scenario. Understanding leads to beauty, which leads to this person having a greater hobby of himself, his capabilities, and what makes him first-rate. Knowing this can help him in finding his strong point and becoming greater rich later in existence.

Chapter 6: You are looking for something new, different, or intriguing?

There is no one like the other. Each of us has different hair colors and skin tones. Some differences are greater than others. Wait, what?

For example, consider hair color. Even though our hair colors might be slightly different, if I have dark hair and you have light hair, it doesn't seem strange to us. Consider a blonde person coming to visit us. Again, the color isn't unusual but different.

These differences can be in hair color, weight, or height. We get used to them over time.

But imagine if we ever see someone with naturally coloured hair. Green? Green? It's strange.

But why is green hair unusual? Because nobody has it.

It is the same for height. Person 10 feet tall would not be just different, he would also be quite unusual.

Why am i mentioning this?

Because scientists are keen to learn about human traits that may be outside the norm. While we may find them odd, an investigator finds them fascinating.

Actually, it would be interesting to meet someone 10 feet tall with green hair. We'd like to find out why this person is different and how it impacts his life.

Perhaps we will one day wish that we could be taller than 10 feet or have more green hair. We might find it attractive to be strange.

What is a "Syndrome"?

A syndrome can be described as a combination of unusual features.

These features are unique enough to stand out. These traits are not necessarily related but often occur in the same person.

John Walks, for example, might observe that people with green hair typically have four fingers on each foot. This is very strange.

John believes the same. He stops and rationalizes, "I don't know what to do. But there seems to be some connection between green hair & feet with four toes." Maybe they are both related to a single gene. John decides that he will look more closely at this group.

Over time, he discovers something extraordinary: they all share a third trait. They all have the ability to quickly get their driver's licence. It's almost as if they were born with the gift to drive vehicles. They are able to climb in and drive a car like they have been doing this for their entire lives.

These days, things are more fascinating than ever. John decides to submit research for publication in a scientific journal.

John starts receiving emails from researchers around world a few days after the publication. He was amazed to discover that many others were also intrigued by the green-haired and four toed individuals. However, they didn't know there a connection to their ability to learn quickly and to be able to drive fast.

John Walks' discovery was greeted with surprise by doctors, scientists, as well as other researchers all over the world who now refer to this bizarre set of 3 traits as "Walks' Syndrome".

Asperger's Syndrome

Hans Asperger, who lived between 1906 - 1980, was for twenty-eight years in charge of the University of Vienna's Pediatrics department. Asperger noticed differences in children through his observations. These differences are however quite strange.

What were the differences?

For instance, he noticed that some children had trouble getting along with others their age. Hans Asperger was intrigued by the normal intelligence of these children. Asperger was actually intrigued by these children because they could talk with him about any subject that interested them and then explain it in detail.

Asperger found that these young boys had difficulties understanding non-verbal communication after examining them more closely. They seemed to be focusing on what they hear, regardless of body language and tone of voice. Additionally, they were slow to express empathy and interest in others.

Hans Asperger contributed more than 300 scientific articles, many of them on autism, to his observations. However, Asperger's research was not acknowledged until his passing.

Today, researchers are still fascinated by these bizarre traits first described by Hans. After Hans Asperger's original work, many scientists started to think that those with these characteristics were "Asperger's Syndrome."

Hans Asperger wasn't the only one to notice these characteristics. Although other researchers also made mention of these traits, none of them achieved the same popularity as Hans Asperger.

Asperger's is a mild form of autism.

What is autism exactly?

my book on safe supplementation of high doses with vitamin D or vitamin K2 describes how the brain is made up billions and trillions of cells that specialize at processing information. These cells are called neuronal. The brain is a company . Each member can be considered a neuron. Each neuron in the brain is a module. Just like employees are assigned to departments, so too is every employee. What way?

An example of a large company's marketing department would include a customer support department, human resources department, and a marketing department. Similar to our brain, there are areas that specialize in processing sound, areas that determine whether the sounds came from other people, or from another source, as well as areas that decipher verbal messages.

A second fascinating area is responsible for extracting subtle messages through the tone of voice, facial expressions, and other human interactions.

Consider this: Imagine approaching a friend and asking them how they are doing. One person might reply with "Hello, how're you?" Is he being honest or just saying "Thank you,"? It depends.

It is important to pay close attention not only to his words but also to his facial expressions and tone. Have you noticed that he spoke slowly, at a low level, and shook his head? If he does this, you will know he's not okay. What's the end result? As a friend, you will adapt your words accordingly.

Next question: "I notice you're feeling ill today. What's the matter?" The person will then vent and feel relieved.

If he had used a bright tone and smiled a lot, it would be easy to believe that he was speaking truthfully.

While you might not have realized it, all this information is stored in your brain. This all happened automatically. You didn't need to keep thinking about this, which would have been a waste of your mental energy. You were able to read his nonverbal cues at any moment. Why? Because autism doesn't exist.

Different brains are autistic. How much different? It's because the brains of autistic people don't develop in areas like communication, socialization, or emotional processing. A person with autism has difficulty processing information such as subtle facial expressions and small variations in volume, tone or voice.

The Autistic Spectrum

Autism exists on a spectrum. This means that someone may be more autistic or less.

Aspergers syndrome is a mild form of autism. This means that someone with Aspergers syndrome may have difficulty understanding the nonverbal messages hidden behind simple statements like "I'm fine. Thank you."

It might take him some time to put this "I'm good, thanks" in context. He will compare it with similar expressions he has heard all his life. He must take the time to reflect on the true meaning of the words that he hears.

But, sometimes an autistic person is too busy to think about it properly and has to risk a reaction. He may think that the person is honest so he doesn't bother to ask "What's up?" Because he didn't pick up the depressing tone,

However, the other person views this indifference in contempt and concludes that autistic people are cold and disinterested. This is not true. The result was simply the result a different brain.

Let's go back to Temple Grandin's analogy. It's as though a customer support department keeps receiving complaints about their product. Yet, nobody seems to care. No spokesperson is available to apologize to the press. The company doesn't react. The company fails to respond. Buyers feel cheated and think that managers of the company don't care enough about their customers.

What's really going on? It turned out that customer service is not communicating the complaints with the company's direction. The direction does not have an accurate idea of how serious the problem is.

Not all autism is the same. A deeper form of autism may be experienced by some people.

They may not even be able react to stimuli outside. As if the customer support department didn't exist, we can go back to our analogy. All complaints end up in the mailboxes.

Autism, however, doesn't affect just communication and social intelligence. These are its most well-known traits because they are the easiest for external observers to see.

What about other areas that are affected? These include those related the processing sensory information, such the temperature perception, as well as areas related to impulse controller, which we will explore in the next chapters.

However, some areas in processing music theory, mathematics, art, and design, as well comprehension and production of written materials, might have evolved beyond the norm.

This could be Asperger's or a milder type of autism. Your child might have someone who plays the piano and composes music, but can't tell the difference between irony and sincerity.

How common is autism?

Today, 1 in 68 individuals is diagnosed with autism. Boys are 4 times more affected by autism than girls.

Researchers however believe that the true number may be greater. Why?

Moderate autism is often not recognized due to its inherent nature. While the rare traits of autism may not be noticed, they are often mistaken for more well-known disorders. They are often encouraged by it. How?

Asperger's syndrome can make it more difficult for someone to feel depressed. This is due to the difficulty in processing emotional information. Sometimes, depression can be diagnosed but not autism. In these cases, the person does not respond to treatment.

Asperger's syndrome often hides the wizard of Oz. However, it can be treated. First, we must recognize it.

You might not be certain of the diagnosis you have or that your child has. Although you notice certain traits, you don't know much about the rest. How can this be solved? It is as simple as abandoning the old ways of thinking.

New way to see autism

We will not be looking at symptoms in this book. Instead we will be looking at the inside of an autistic brain.

This will allow us all to learn how to best deal with the autistic personality.

This is why this approach is better

As an example, let's say your child is hypersensitive to sensory stimuli. This refers to hypersensitivity in the brain that is involved with processing one or more sensory inputs.

This might be the only sign your child may have, aside from minor difficulties with social interaction. If this is true, your child won't be given an autism diagnosis. The problem of hypersensitivity persists, and you must know how to deal with it.

With the right knowledge about autism, it's possible to see the hidden message behind bizarre behaviors like stimming. These are the repetitive and unusual movements that define autism.

An autism specialist, you

The best way to become an autism specialist is to learn how to handle each of these autistic traits.

These symptoms aren't unusual, but they will be fascinating to you.

It doesn't matter what type of trait or degree. When you know what's happening, you'll be able deal with any trait, no matter how severe.

It could be you or your child, your student, a coworker, or anyone else. You'll quickly recognize a behavior and be able to determine how to respond. It is easy to do this with the right tools.

Even if you're the autistic one, it still applies. This book will give you a fresh perspective on your life.

Imagine looking back at yourself and saying, "Oh! So that's Why I ...""" Or: "Now I understand!" This is why I behaved as this when...

A book like this will give you the knowledge you need to make better decisions. Make decisions that are beneficial for you and others with autism, including those you care about. By doing so, you can better predict what the future holds, which behaviors will lead to meltdowns, and how to make better decisions.

It will also be easier to tell the difference between bad advice and good advice.

Chapter 7: What is the Autistic Brain's Work Process?

People are more attractive at a bar. Why?

Because alcohol is known to cause a disruption in the area that is responsible for detecting symmetry in people's faces.

The right side of someone's face should look the same as the one on the left. This makes them more attractive. This makes sense. It makes sense. Same goes for the nose, mouth and all other aspects of the human body.

How is this assessment done?

There is a part of our brain that responds to this question when we are looking at the faces of another person.

There are 10 possible answers to this question: What is the degree symmetry of the person's face, from 0 to 10?

If the answer is 10, the brain will perceive the person as beautiful. The influence on our perception of beauty will be much less if the answer is 0. How does alcohol influence this process?

You can make your brain give 10 to anyone who drinks too much alcohol.

However, that is not the only effect alcohol has on the brain.

A person who drinks excessive alcohol has a negative effect on their motor coordination, reasoning, ability to avoid reactions and self-control. It's unreasonable to expect someone who is drunk to be able maintain an intelligent conversation or walk straight.

This example shows that there are many areas in our brains and that when one is affected, it affects our entire set of abilities and personality.

How does this relate with autism?

chapter 1. - We briefly looked at how autistic individuals can't recognize facial expressions and tone of voice. Let's look into this concept more deeply.

One brain, many specialized area

Our brain has a great task at any given moment: keeping us connected to the real-world. This involves the processing of sensory stimuli as well as deciding what information is important and what information is not.

Your brain must also be aware of other cars and obstacles when driving your car.

Imagine you're driving down the road when you see the driver in front of your suddenly apply the brakes. Although you may have been distracted, you will be able to see that the brake lights are activated. Instantly your heart starts to beat faster, your blood pressure rises, and your hands start to get cold. However, this sudden burst can allow you to quickly react, slow down your vehicle, and avoid hitting other drivers.

The entire process took only a few seconds, but required the processing of huge amounts of information. It was a simple task of slowing down your car. But it required coordination across your entire brain.

Let's look closer at this process. We'll be done and you will have learned something about autism. Prepared?

Communication -- The basis of mental processing

Your brain began to chat with the front cars when they turned on the red lights. It asked questions and responded to each one. Let us simplify the matter by visualizing all of your brain's areas video conferencing with one other.

Visual perception: The red lights are lit up. What does this signify?"

Area responsible for comparing real-life events with our past memories.

Decision-Making Zone: "What should you do?"

Area responsible for comparing real-world events with our past memories.

Decision-Making Zone: "Which is the best option?"

Area responsible for comparing real-life events with our past memories. Braking is better.

Decision-Making Area: "How do we brake? "

Area responsible to compare what's happening in real life with our memories of the past: "You must press the center pedal with the right foot as hard you can."

Decision-Making area: "Roger That, I'm transferring all this information into the conscious mind for prompt implementation."

Now, consider what was happening while you were driving the car.

You noticed that the lights were on. A few moments later, your conscious awareness brought up the idea of moving the left foot towards the center pedal. This was your only responsibility.

Let's look closer at the dialogue. It is possible to imagine the same dialogue taking place in a driving course.

The student sits at the wheel of the car for the first-time. He seems to be moving slowly, but all of it seems to catch his attention. He is travelling at 20 mph but the car in front brakes abruptly. "What now?" "What now?" he asks his instructor. "Now brake!" You must press the accelerator fast! The instructor replies.

After a few weeks, he had his driver's license and was driving his own vehicle. He no longer needs an instructor telling him what to go do. But he still needs time to process the information.

He thinks to himself while pressing down on the central accelerator.

In the initial weeks of his license, he may be too focused on his driving that he cannot have a conversation. He will improve as he gets more experience.

His brain is familiar with driving now that he has been driving for a few more months. He's able to adapt to new situations. He may never have had to deal with an animal crossing his street. He doesn't have time to think about what happens when that happens. He feels compelled to brake immediately. This urge is so strong and so intense that he can't help wanting to brake as quickly as possible.

However, do you recall the first conversation he had avec his instructor? It's still there. It became automatic, unconscious.

Congratulations.

Now you know something fundamental. What?

You didn't get a brain that was capable of driving a car. You had to learn how to do this. The initial process was tiring. Everything was new when you first sat in the driver's seat.

Your communication with your instructor was essential. He gave you the instructions, the how-to, and the when.

"Now shift gears. You will need to press the left pedal using your left foot. As long as the pedal is not down, move your shift lever backwards and to the side.

However, what if your driving instructor instead of taking you step-by-step through the process, and simply said "Let's go to home"?

You would reply, "But I've never driven before. I don't even know how the car should be started. I need specific instructions.

If we need to complete a task and have not had our brains prepared for it from birth, we need specific instructions.

Do you remember the green-haired patients with the syndrome we created earlier? People with Walk's syndrome had 4 toes right on their right feet, green hair and were very good drivers.

These people were born with brains that are multi-functional and capable of driving. Scientists have no idea why but Walks' patients have an entire area dedicated to steering. Another area is dedicated to processing information related the use and operation of the pedals. The shift lever is also covered in 2 separate areas. It seems like magic. But, when you put someone with Walks' Syndrome in a vehicle, he looks like a fish in water. He is at ease. His hands and feet move to all the right spots. It's amazing to witness. It looks like he has been doing this all his life.

Now, imagine that someone with Walks' syndrome is trying teach someone else how it feels to drive. What would their dialogue look like? Let's see.

Person with Walks' syndrome - "Okay, now please let's start our car and drive around the neighbourhood."

Common person:

"What is Person with Walks' Syndrome?" The car is turned on and that's it.

For now, this is the end. You might not be aware of it, but you have learned more about autism over the course of your life than most people. Let's now look at the essential truths about autism we have discovered so far.

The brains of autistic people don't have fully developed neurological connections to empathy, interpretations of nonverbal communication and socialization. For him, it's like learning to drive a car. But this "car", however, has thousands upon thousands of buttons!

This is in contrast to those who are not autistic and can drive a car from birth.

An autistic person is also known as a neurotypical. This is someone whose brain displays a typical or common neurological configuration. Neurotypicals don't understand how this happens. However, their "hands-and-feet," which refers to his body language, facial expressions, words and body language, simply "travel" all the way. His brain is capable of processing all the necessary information unconsciously since birth. This allows him to make friends and communicate with people.

What can you do to help the autistic improve their social skills? You can see how this is not possible in the dialog below.

Neurotypical person: Please make friends at school.

Autistic person says, "But, how can I make friends?"

Neurotypical person: You meet the people and then become friends.

Can you see the frustration that each one of them must feel after this discussion?

The neurotypical person is unable to comprehend how such a simple task could be so difficult. It's quite simple. "You get there, you say hello, and everything flows naturally."

However, even if the neurotypical person attempted to explain, he would have difficulty explaining each step. Why? Because social interaction is part of his nature. His brain has many dedicated areas that can perform numerous processes at the unconscious and conscious levels.

How can the neurotypical examine his unconscious and figure out how to help someone with different abilities? It's like asking an Englishman for help teaching his language to a Portuguese speaker. The first place to look is the one you are in. This is not an easy task unless the Englishman speaks English fluently. For him, English speaking comes as a natural ability.

For autistic individuals, however, the situation can be more frustrating. Depending upon the severity of autism, the idea of making friends may be as difficult or as simple as driving a commercial aircraft. If an autistic person is close to another person, it can feel like they are in the cockpit of the Boeing A320.

He keeps trying hard to remember what to say: "Okay. First I say, "Hi, how're you?" I wait for an answer and then I say... Then, I wait for the answer.

The problem is worse because even if he knows everything, social interactions are unpredictable.

The person with autism responds by saying "Hi, how are your days?" But his facial expressions and tone of voice are not the best. It's as though he's in the cockpit of an aircraft, pressing the wrong button but holding the correct lever. Any competent pilot would instantly realize that he was a beginner. The children in the same way realize that there is something wrong with their "Hi, how are your?"

How can I help someone with autism

We'll return to our example of the driving class. The instructor may not immediately show you how to drive a car. He will only teach you the basics. You learn that your car can't hit other cars. You discover which foot corresponds with which pedal, as well as other simple rules. However, it is only when you are actually driving that you really begin to understand the workings of everything.

This teaches you that it is possible to violate the traffic law if a car is blocking the roadway. To avoid an obstacle, you may need breaking the rule not to step on a continuously white line.

These situations offer the instructor the chance to show you practical applications of the driving code. This will give you a deeper learning experience.

Soon you will be able see the big picture and understand how to deal with a completely different situation.

This holds true for any task you need to complete that you do not have specialized knowledge in.

We were not created with the brains to drive cars or change a burning light bulb.

Each of these cases requires us to be instructed, step by step. This instruction must be specific, clear and simple. We can only get a sense of the tasks involved if we do it ourselves. The more times you do it, the more different situations there will be. As we become more proficient at dealing with these situations, we gain greater proficiency in the task.

If you have been involved in building walls for more than 30 years under adverse conditions and have laid bricks over the same period, you can be confident that you are ready to handle any new situations. You are an expert.

This task required constant conscious effort from the beginning: "Which brick shall I grab first?" How much mortar should you use? Which place should I lay this brick in? How much pressure should I put on this new brick to match the rest?

It's 30 years later, and all of this dialogue occurs automatically in your mind. You don't even know that it exists. If the wall starts to bend towards one side, you will automatically know what to go. Even if you have to stop and think about how to solve a problem that presents itself, the majority of processing occurs in your unconscious.

You were not born with a brain that is specialized in building walls. However, with lots of practical experience and time you have developed a "pseudo"-area. But how? It turns out, that other areas of your being -- such as motor coordination and abstract thinking, color perception, distance perception, and mathematical calculation, among others -- have learned how to work together so you can lay bricks like no-one else.

This is exactly the case with autism.

When the autistic brain is required to perform a task for a task for that which he does not have a specialized area, he must be taught each step. These steps must be simple and specific, as in the instruction manual for washing machines. This manual was intended to be helpful for someone who had never used a washing machine.

How do you teach autistic brains anything?

You will need to provide simple instructions for more complicated tasks.

The autistic person must have many opportunities to experiment and get feedback about how he can improve.

He needs someone to assist him in understanding that the "brick is not well placed." That is not all. He needs a specialist to show him the correct way to place the brick. This information must be presented in simple and clear language.

There are many parts of the autistic brain which don't function well. However, there are still other areas that work perfectly. Some of them even work well. This means they must understand the instructions.

The areas of abstract thinking are not good examples. This is why you must speak clearly. This is critical. It's the first.

What is the distinction between concrete and abstract language. How can you ensure you are communicating with an autistic brain in a manner he understands? This is the next chapter.

Chapter 8: The Difference between Concrete and Abstract Thinking -- The Secret of Communicating With Someone with Autism

Autism suffers from difficulties processing abstract language. Concrete language is easy to process. Concrete language is a great way to communicate with Asperger's or moderate autism.

If you are trying to communicate with someone with more severe autism, be aware that his or her communication centres may be completely disabled. Concrete language is the best way to communicate with someone with autism.

What is concrete speech?

You can point to something concrete. These are things that can be referred to. They can all be touched, smelled and felt.

What about abstract language, though?

Take a look at these examples of abstract thought:

"Dogs, are mammals."

"We have to love each other."

"It is good to be alive."

"Dogs, are mammals"

These sentences are immediately understood by a neurotypical individual who has read them.

Autism sufferers must be able to translate abstract ideas into concrete concepts. Then, he can understand. This process is nearly automatic but it is still possible for autistic people.

"Dogs," and "mammals," are categories that can be referred to as concepts, but not things like bread and water.

Please note this comment from someone who has autism

To understand the abstract concept of "dogs", in my case my brain immediately shows me images of different breeds of dogs. It happens so fast that it is almost impossible to miss. Same goes for the word "mammals". Instantly, I think of a whale jumping and leaving behind water. Next, I imagine an image featuring many other mammal animals, such as bears, seals, and dolphins. If I ask my brain "What is mammal?" My brain says that mammals are animals that are born to drink milk. >>

Did you notice the pattern. The Asperger's man needed something tangible to help him understand the abstract concept "mammal". He also needed a definition of the word, which used concrete ideas like milk, in order to define it.

If this conversion is not possible, the meaning of the word "mammal," will cease to be meaningful for an autistic person.

The better he understands the boundaries of a given category by seeing more examples (mammals, clothing, subcategories, dogs, etc.

Abstract thinking can be learned from a young age. The word "mammal", when you hear it, you instantly know what it means. You don't have to look for concrete things like "pictures" (or "definitions that include concrete explanations).

Unbelieving the differences between abstract and concrete thinking, an Asperger's patient said:

I didn't even know this abstract thinking existed. It's hard to imagine how something can be understood without concrete examples. >>

Notice how this man describes his mental processes in order to understand "possible", for example.

I notice the image of someone reaching out to grab something. He is trying get something. I have an image of someone jumping off the edge of a rock to try to reach the other side. This helps me to better understand the meaning. My brain basically gives me

87

concrete images and videos to help me understand the abstract concept that is "possible". >>

The images that come up in an autistic mind may not all make sense to everyone else. Some are images mixed in with emotions, and some appear very quickly. However, their brain needs to find something palpable it already knows well to understand abstract languages.

It's as though the abstract concept is the roof, while the concrete concepts are the walls, pillars and other supporting foundations.

"We have got to love one other."

It is the same with "We have to Love One Another."

Again, we reach out to Aspergers, who chose to remain anonymous and asked him for his thoughts.

To me, the phrase "love one another" doesn't mean anything. I don't understand what it means to say that you have to love me. In my mind, I automatically see the image of someone hugging another or of one person offering something to another. >>

What is "love?" Only by combining all these concrete pictures can the autistic mind come to a conclusion.

However, this conclusion only applies to the concrete examples the autistic person is able to see.

The more concrete examples that he has, both his understanding and his ability to recognize whether a new action falls within the definition of "loving others" will increase.

Let's say, for example, that we ask this person to "Is shaking hands part 'loving people?'" This is a fascinating explanation.

I can picture two people shaking hands when I think about being in love. They are wearing a suit and an combining tie. They are smiling and shaking hands. One holds the other's hand. You can tell they are good friends. You can love other people by shaking hands. >>

The neurotypical individual doesn't require this intermediate step, as his brain already understands the concept of "loving another".

"It is good to be alive."

The expression, "It's good being alive" is a similar one. I am reminded of the image above: a smiling person sitting. The camera then turns its attention to his breathing. The person is smiling while keeping his eyes closed. He also takes deep breaths. "Good" is a picture of someone smiling, which helps me to understand the meanings of individual words in the sentence. "Alive", makes a little video of someone breathing. If I look at the meaning of "alive", an image of someone in a chair appears with a comment: "It is the opposite of that." >>

These concrete examples are not always the same. However, this doesn't necessarily mean these videos or images will never appear. But something concrete will happen in the autistic mind.

One thing is constant: an autistic brain cannot understand abstract concepts unless it has concrete examples to illustrate them. The more concrete examples an autistic person is able to provide, the greater his understanding of abstract concepts.

It's important to explain autism to autistic people by showing them a story or image and saying, "This is an example for "x".

The autistic will eventually understand the meaning "x" when they have seen many examples. How does the person find out if the autistic understands "x"? When he is capable of creating his own completely unique examples for "x".

Let's see an example of the abstract explanation.

What is an abstraction concept?

Every abstract concept has a list of rules that tells it what belongs to it and what doesn't.

These rules are written using concrete language. When they aren't concrete, they are written using an abstract language closer the concrete. It's a bit like an onion. There are several layers of abstraction.

Consider, for example: The word "mammals". Here are some guidelines:

They are vertebrates.

The mammary glands of females produce milk and feed their babies.

Except for the embryonic hair of some whales and dolphins, all animals have fur.

Their heart is made up of four chambers.

The expression "Their four chambers are their heart" is far more abstract than "mammals"

We again turn to someone with autism, to learn how the autistic mind works.

I can easily visualize a heart that has four divisions. Although the word "chambers", though, is not very concrete. I can picture pyramids with many chambers or divisions. Once that is understood, the concept of a heart has four rooms. >>

"Mammary glands" on the other is concrete.

I see a cow with her mammary cells. It's the very first image that comes up in my head. >>

What is the lesson for us all?

You can communicate with someone with autism by giving them as many examples of your own experiences as you can. Use concrete language for these examples. Ask him to make his own examples. Ask him to create some new examples.

He will understand, but you'll be amazed at the mental fluidity he uses to connect his new understanding with everything else and create new ideas.

How can you teach yourself how to make abstract concepts concrete?

Imagine that writing and speaking were your only options. What is the best way to explain an abstract idea in English?

Imagine being able only to explain the meaning of the word "mammal", but without the ability or knowledge to write. What would you do to accomplish this task?

Maybe mimicking. If so, what gestures could you use? To which direction would your point? What would be the first thing you would draw on a piece or paper?

It is likely that you would draw animals. If you could draw only 3 or 4 animals would it be sufficient to explain that you are referring to "mammals", and not to the abstract concept "animals"?

Perhaps you end up drawing other animals than mammals such as birds and fish. Then, put an "X" on it to indicate that they're out.

In reality, it would be like saying:

"These are the limits to the abstract concept I want you learn. "Whales, dogs, cats, and other animals are within their bounds. This sardine is outside the bounds.

But that wouldn't be enough to define the boundaries of "mammal" in any way. It would take many more animals. Many different animal types can be sketched on one sheet of paper. You could make hundreds or even thousands of them. You can describe what you want to explain better if you have more examples.

It would eventually come to a point that the other person would be capable of seeing which animals are included in each category, even if they didn't know you were talking specifically about "mammals".

Try explaining more abstract ideas, such as "category", "abstract" meanings or even "example", and "concept". If you don't speak or write, it becomes more complicated.

Your task will be easier if your level of abstraction is lower and you try to explain simpler abstract terms such as "clothing," "food", or "books".

Therefore, you should start with the concrete. Slowly, move onto the abstract.

Show him pictures from magazines and online, draw pictures or give him objects to help him understand concrete concepts. Use these concrete examples as stepping blocks to teach him abstract concepts. As he learns more, his brain will be able to better understand spoken and written languages.

This means that you'll be teaching "cat", by showing images of cats to your child and repeating "cat!" every time. Your child will be able point to new images of cats and identify them systematically when he can do this. Once he can do that, you can start to teach him new concepts.

Your challenge is greater the higher your level of autism. Some autistic people may need to take longer to learn basic words. Keep trying! You will reap the rewards of your hard work.

Alternativ, you could also ask what you should teach someone with Asperger's who has a moderate level of autism.

Focus your efforts on helping him learn more abstract concepts in the areas that he is most challenged.

In the next chapter we will examine one of the areas where autistic children require the most assistance: the development Emotional Intelligence.

We will explore each of the human fundamental emotions and discuss how we can help autistic persons to be more able to manage them.

These instructions are most useful for individuals with autism who can communicate. However the basic principles will work for all types of autism.

Chapter 9: Emotional Intelligence -- Autism can be used to understand emotions

This chapter was created to explain an abstract concept called emotional intelligence in a concrete manner. You can adapt the chapter to be helpful for someone with autism. The examples should be adjusted to reflect the understanding level and age of the person being taught.

The chapter will also assist autistic individuals in significantly increasing their emotional intelligence.

Even someone with autism can still benefit from the information provided here, as it is universal.

Where should you begin?

We begin with the brain. Our brain has specific areas that help us evaluate our resources and determine our needs.

When one of these changes occurs, our bodies alert us and adapt to the situation.

These two words can confuse you. Don't worry. This will be made clear by the following examples. Next we will discuss autism and how it all fits together.

Not enough

Human needs are the same for everyone. These needs include:

Essen

Drinking water

Sleeping

It is when you take a rest, such as when we lie down for a time to recover our energy.

Breathing

Our bodies should be at the correct temperature

It is important to get away from the things that cause us pain

Excretion

To meet these needs, we use resources.

Resources

A resource is all that is available to meet a particular need. You can use different resources, like bread, meat, rice or fruit and vegetables to satisfy your hunger.

Water is a vital resource for drinking water.

It doesn't matter if we need to sleep. All that matters is that we have the right place to relax and be able sleep comfortably. You need to be able to sit down for a while to get some rest.

For breathing, there is another resource that cannot be replaced: oxygen with the right amount of gases.

Our body needs to be at the correct temperature. There are many resources that can help us do this.

Accessing specific resources like a doctor or medication is essential to getting rid of any pain. We just need enough space for us to move away any potential pain.

To excrete, you need to have adequate sanitation facilities. Or at least an open field.

These are basic needs all of us have. They are also met with resources. There are many other, less tangible needs that we will soon discuss.

Emotions

What happens to our needs if they are not met? Two things will occur:

Your body will tell you when to expect something through sensations.

Our brain will flood our conscious minds with suggestions about what we should do next.

1. Our bodies sends warnings through our senses

Certain areas of the brain are responsible for monitoring our needs. It is complex because they use hormones, electric signals and the interaction of the brain with our organs.

This is how you get the sensation of hunger.

Our brain communicates continuously with the stomach, and all other organs. The brain will eventually get the message: "We need to eat more." All this communication happens in the background without our knowledge. It's an unconscious process.

When the unconscious part sends a message, it makes the person feel hungry. While his thoughts were focused on the work at hand, his brain is now more interested in food.

Our bodies believe we have to eat more, so the greater our hunger and thoughts about food.

The same applies for other needs.

Food = we feel hungry.

Water intake = We feel thirsty.

Sleep = We feel asleep.

Rest = We feel tired.

Breathing = We feel an increasing distress when we are unable or unable to breath, as when we are submerged.

Comfort is when our body is at the right temp.

Removing from things that cause pain = If we ignore these needs, we will feel the pain.

Excretion refers to the desire or need to urinate/defecate.

2. Our brain will flood our conscious minds with suggestions for next steps.

Our brains were able to learn what resources could be used for our needs when we were young. Water is what we look at when we're thirsty.

Food = We tend to think more about food.

Water intake = When we think of drinking water, it is the first thing that comes to our minds.

Sleep = We often think about how nice it would be if we could just lay down on the bed.

Rest = The thoughts we have about how wonderful it would feel to be able to relax keep popping up in our minds.

Breathing = If this need is met, we don't know what else to do. The only thing we care about is how to breathe.

A body that is at the right temperature = Ideas about how to heat us up come up if we are cold. If it is too hot, then we have to think about how to cool off or taking a shower.

Staying away from things that cause you pain = If we touch something that causes discomfort, our first instinct is to move on. Our minds fill up with ideas of how we can escape. If we are convinced that something could hurt us, our minds can only think about how we can escape it.

Excretion = Our thoughts are limited to the toilet. If the need becomes too overwhelming, more bold ideas may come to our minds, such as urinating in a bush.

Let's now move onto the abstract. Prepared?

Depending on the beliefs we hold about the resources available to us, we may feel an emotion.

Let's take a look at the meaning of the phrase. It is important to discuss the emotions our bodies experience.

There are many ways to describe emotions. Paul Ekman, an expert in emotion research, says that there are just a few basic emotions. These emotions can combine with others and create complex emotions.

What are our fundamental, or primary emotions?

Happiness

Fear

Anger

Disgust

Surprise

Sadness

Let us now look at each one. Don't despair. You will see the difference in just a few minutes. In a matter of minutes, you will have concrete information that will make a difference in people's lives. This will enable your to easily understand and explain all of the abstract worlds of needs, resources and emotions.

Find the pattern and see if you can spot it.

Understanding the Emotions and Happiness

We are content when we know we have a resource that can fulfill our needs. And then we are happy when it is actually used to satisfy our needs.

Examples:

I'm hungry. I remember the delicious dish that my wife cooked for me. I feel happy. I smell the food as soon as I get back home. My expectation of being met soon grows. My happiness is greater. I sit down at my table and begin to eat. I feel satisfied after finishing the meal. This satisfaction is what we refer to as happiness. It's more that a single moment of joy, laughter or even a feeling of contentment. These are just a few examples.

I'm sleepy. I imagine that at the end the day, I will have a comfortable place to sleep. I go to sleep when it's night. I feel happy whenever I wake up, because I satisfied my sleeping need.

The same thing happens when we breathe deeply and when we finally forget about the pain.

Wrap yourself in a warm blanket when you feel cold.

When we are tired, finally sit down.

When we're in desperate need of the bathroom, but the toilet is occupied. The door suddenly opens and allows us to enter. We feel happy.

Happiness is measured in degrees. Higher levels of happiness are associated with greater certainty about my ability to satisfy my needs. The remaining emotions will be discussed next.

What is the purpose and meaning of happiness?

Happiness can be a motivating factor. It encourages us to make use of the resources that satisfy our needs. We will be more likely to return to that resource for our next needs.

Understanding Fear

Fear can be caused by the belief that something will happen to a resource which meets a specific need. Many changes occur in the body when this expectation is realized. These sensations are called fear. This combination of sensations, changes, and fear is what we call "fear."

Imagine, for example, that my boss calls and asks me to meet in his office. His voice sounds irritated and tense. I think back on the mistakes that I made last week. Will I be lectured about my mistakes? Will I get fired?

I am more likely to believe these outcomes than I am to fear.

But why are I afraid? Because I am certain that I need my job to be able access to the resources necessary to meet my needs. My job is what gives me the money I need to eat and provides food.

The value I feel I have from this job is also higher. My job is my value. Why is value important? It is fascinating that "value", in ancient Greek, was linked to the concept of weight. The smaller my "value" in comparison to other people's, the greater the "weight" that I need for them. I will have less influence over their decisions and ability to deal with them.

When I was faced with the possibility to lose my job, my brain kept thinking about all of these possibilities. This is how we experience fear and the emotions that accompany it.

Another example is the health. I may google for the symptoms of a heart attack if I have chest pains. I read on about the signs of imminent heart attacks, such as chest pains, fatigue, difficulty breathing, and "chest pains". What is the result? The outcome?

In these cases, fear does not seem useful. How does fear stop me being fired from my job? How can fear prevent me from having a cardiac attack?

But the truth is that fear can be very helpful. Fear is for protection. Fear can make us more vigilant and more likely to take the right decisions.

For example, if feeling confident, I'll speak to my boss differently than if it is scary. Fear will help me be careful, acknowledge my mistake, and apologize.

The symptoms of a heartattack are the same. Fear will motivate me to do something. Call 911, drive to the hospital.

Imagine, as the last example: you're out walking along the street when a large dog approaches. The dog is huge and it's barking at the passerby. He moves towards you and growls at you. Your brain is unsure how to respond so it quickly calculates "This dog may attack me." The greater your fear, the more likely you are to believe (1) you can be attacked or (2) that this attack could cause serious injury. The greater your fear, the more focused you are on doing everything possible to protect yourself.

Depending upon what you believe to the right thing, fear might cause you to stay still and paralyzed, not to move, or even to attack the dog.

What is the purpose and function of fear?

Fear is the term for the emotions that we feel in our bodies when there is a threat. Fear makes it clear that we won't ignore this threat, and that we will do whatever we can to make it through it. The beliefs we hold about the situation will influence what actions we take.

Understanding Emotions: Anger

Anger is one the most intriguing emotions for me. When we believe in injustice, anger is a natural emotion. We feel the need to seek justice so much that we have a whole emotion for dealing with any attack on our beliefs about fairness.

Anger is a very powerful emotion. Our brain emits many hormones and messengers when it senses an injustice. Which way?

Our conscious mind is full of thoughts about how injustice could be corrected. We feel our heart beating fast, our breathing gets faster, and our muscles become tighter. This is why? Because our brain has turned our entire body into war machines.

If anger isn't controlled it can cause a lot of damage. It can lead us into doing things that we regret.

However, anger in and of itself is not evil.

Like fear, anger drives us to action. The problem is that anger can sometimes become overwhelming and difficult to manage. Consider anger as a fast vehicle. Your speed will determine how long it takes to halt and change the direction. Also, it is difficult to stay away from violent thoughts when you are angry. All because our brain sensed injustice.

What is an injustice?

"Injustice," is an abstract term. How can we make it more concrete? Imagine a judge. The judge's job is directly linked to justice.

Judges make a comparison between the two sides of a case. Judges make a comparison of what should happen and what actually occurred. The judge then makes a decision about what should be done. To reach that conclusion, the judge must consider the intent of those who have committed the wrong act.

As an example, suppose that an elderly lady is walking down the street when she drops her wallet. How should other people respond? The best thing to do is pick up the wallet, call her and give it back. This means that a woman who grabs the wallet and places it in her pocket is wrong.

This judge is faced with the situation and compares what was done -- taking the wallet -- to what should have happened: returning the wallet.

If the wallet were returned, the judge might have ruled that it was fair. The judge would be content, and he would commend the man for being honest. The wallet was stolen. This is an injustice. This should not have happened. It angered the judge and he felt the need to reestablish law.

The judge will then consider the appropriate course. He may decide that the lady should be compensated for all her anxiety and the money she lost. He may also decide that the thief is guilty of wrongdoing.

But before the judge makes his final decision the judge will take into consideration the intent of each man. This could make all the difference.

Imagine, for example that several eyewitnesses testify the man was nearly ready to return the wallet. However, he didn't because of circumstances beyond the man's control. Although the outcome of the case is the same, the judge's opinions change. After the judge recognizes that the man had good intentions, he ceases feeling angry. Perhaps he is feeling sad now as he considers the emotional turmoil the whole situation has caused to both the man, and to the elderly lady.

Our brain also has many rules that describe what we believe right and wrong.

While we may not think much about it, justice is something that every human being must seek. This is a trait that children are exposed to early. Children find it unfair when their schoolmate has a bigger piece of cake than they do.

It's fascinating to think about how even a burglar can sense justice. The thief isn't happy to be robbed. He gets furious. His brain keeps telling him, "It's not fair!" He becomes angry at the one who stole from him.

Anger drives action. For the child, anger can lead to him crying or demanding an explanation. In the case the thief he might plot to exact his revenge.

Anger is the inner force that makes us feel angry and pushes us to make things right. This inner force arises when our brain, acting like a judge compares what happened to what we think should have occurred. If there is any difference between these things, and if it seems that the other person has bad intentions, our brain creates an image of an enemy. We get angry.

Sometimes we can even become angry at ourselves. This happens when we realize what we should have done. However, this is not a common situation where we would use "anger". Some people use other expressions, such as "I am annoyed by myself" or "I'm so frustrated at me." However, they all refer to the exact same emotion, anger, but in a greater or lesser extent.

What is the purpose and effect of anger?

Anger can lead to impatience. We want to make things right. Unfortunately, anger blinds us. It drives us to act but doesn't tell what to do. People with bad morals or little self-control may end up hurting others. When used appropriately, anger is a powerful motivator for us to act in a constructive direction.

If I witness a lady being robbed and am angry, I will want to do something to help the lady. For example, I might call the cops and wait for the lady to calm down before calling the police. I felt angry or outraged. This strong emotion kept my hands from being indifferent and allowing me to do nothing.

Understanding Emotions

Our physical and mental energy are the most important resources that we have. Because of this, our brain is wired to want to keep us from being exhausted mentally or physically.

Consider, for example, what happens if you ask me to perform some calculations?

Take the test.

$1 + 1 = ?$

$3 + 5 = ?$

$24 + 65 = ?$

$55 + 15 = ?$

$9 \times 78 = ?$

$1849 \times 4, = ?$

$354651 - 456651 = ?$

$2375 / 51 = ?$

Did you notice it? Your brain became less capable of solving complicated problems. You felt disgusted. Unless you have plenty of mental energy. Continue solving complex problems if this is the case. Soon your body is going to warn you about the decrease in mental energy. What's the solution?

If you don't like math, your stomach will tighten and muscles will tighten. If you hate math you might feel nausea.

We are used to thinking of disgust as the smell of rotten food, or the sight of a disturbing picture. However, disgust can be used as a general protection mechanism.

Our unconscious mind is constantly deciding whether a stimulus will be too much for our body. If it is then, we modify our body to make it less difficult to reject it. How can you demonstrate this?

Here's another example: spoiled foods. If you smell rotten food, you will feel your body constrict. Instead of preparing your body for digestion, your digestive system will begin to work to expell the food.

Of course, we don't always realize that other people or objects can also cause that same emotion. The problem is that just like our bodies have trouble digesting spoiled food our minds also have trouble processing interaction with difficult people.

Our minds can become exhausted from dealing with complicated people. It is not surprising that even the thought of spending one afternoon with one these people can affect our health. It was as if our brain was telling us our body is refusing to deal the person with the exact same intensity it rejects spoiled foods.

Sometimes just being tired can be enough. If we're tired, the mere thought of solving 41 + 27, can make our stomachs turn in disgust.

Can you recall a time that you didn't want to be around anyone? Perhaps you were tired from a hard day's work, or maybe you were just feeling tired. These are times when even the thought of dealing with a loved ones can cause some level of disgust.

At these times, it feels as if our brain is constantly telling us "I refuse processing more information!" I want to relax!

The more that we believe that something will bring us down, then the more disgusting we will feel.

What is the purpose and function of disgust?

Disgust allows us to refuse things that make us miserable or harm us. It's only a protection mechanism. It is a motivator to stay away from these types of stimuli.

Understanding Emotions is a Surprise

Our brains are very fast. It processes huge amounts of information at all times. Our brain is not infinitely quick.

Imagine yourself about to enter your home and open the door after a hard day's work. As you open the door to your home, your brain is working overtime to assist. Details about what you have to do next will appear in your brain. Imagine yourself entering the house, turning on the lights, putting your keys, coat, and keys in the correct place, then walking to the bathroom to wash and refresh your skin.

When you are done with the key-locking and rolling of the key, the actions will all flow easily, almost in sync. You don't have to use mental energy. Your home is your mental refuge and your source of relaxation. But...

Imagine how you feel when you turn on your light. Everything is upside down. The drawers open. The furniture is dispersed all over. You can see the papers and clothes scattered about. What do your thoughts? How do you feel?

After a while, you will be still. Take the time to process all that you have just noticed.

Your brain is unable to process the situation in real time because it has encountered something completely different. It takes just a couple of seconds. You are feeling surprised.

Surprise is an emotion when the unexpected happens. Our brains and bodies adapt to the new situation.

Take a look at these examples:

While you are focused on a task at hand, your cell phone rings. For a brief moment, you become paralyzed and change the "disk" in your brain.

Crossing the road is a way of asking yourself what you will do when getting to the shop. Instantly, you hear the sound of rubber fighting asphalt. Your body becomes paralysed and your brain is unable to process what is happening. Do I run or jump? Do I run, or jump? You finally decide which option is best.

When you're speaking to your wife, suddenly her face becomes pale. You stand there paralyzed. "What happened?" Finally you murmur "What happened?"

You find yourself in a foreign place and suddenly, someone shouts your name.

These examples demonstrate the important point: When our brain processes something unexpectedly that it considers urgent, all other mental functions are put on hold.

One could even argue that surprise is a "preemotion" in the sense that it occurs before other emotions. It is the instant before the brain decides how it should respond.

Sometimes, though, this moment can last longer than a few minutes.

Recall our example. After gazing for a few seconds at the chaos in your house, you finally stop processing this unsettling situation. "I have been robbed."

What will it be like to feel next? It depends. Fear is when you feel that thieves may be still in your home or you fear they might rob you again. Anger can also be experienced as you realise the severity of the situation. Sometimes you may feel severe pain in the stomach when your mind grasps how absurd this is. You may feel strong feelings of disgust in this situation.

"Call 911, get help, look for the culprits, and grieve the loss.

This trial may lead to some people literally vomiting from disgust.

What is the purpose and function of surprise?

Our bodies respond to surprise by processing information more quickly. Our previous thoughts remain in the background as we stand still. Our body is alert and ready to react when the situation presents itself.

In the meantime, the brain analyzes how the situation changes our resources and their needs. Then, it decides on the appropriate emotion.

Understanding the Emotions

Sadness and loss are intimately linked. People, for example are a resource to meet our needs. You might find this sentence cold. If so, you should consider the following:

Human beings have a fundamental need to help others. We can do this because we have the support of other people. By doing so, they become a resource which allows us to fulfill our desire for their well-being.

Let's discuss happiness again. We feel happy when we can meet our needs. This is how the brain rewards us when our needs are met. Let's ask the question: Which makes us happier? Meeting our own needs or those of others?

These situations are possible to imagine:

I have a loaf. There is a hungry child in front. I can even see his silhouette. I could be hungry. Eating bread would satisfy me and provide some satisfaction. How would I feel eating bread with a hungry child staring at me? Would I feel truly happy? But what if I gave my child all the bread? My joy will be so intense that I might find myself with tears in my eyes.

Some videos captured by security cameras at train stations show people who, inadvertently or otherwise, fall into the train tracks. What is the reaction of other people? They take risks by helping others get out of trouble. They may feel a little guilty when they look back at what they did. Happy, satisfied.

A parent who cares about their child offers to donate organs, such as a part of their liver or a kidney.

To love others more, it's easier to put their needs first than ours. When we do that, we feel great satisfaction.

By doing so, others can become a resource that meets our needs.

As you can see this is very traumatizing. The loss of a loved one means that we cannot contribute to their well being. It takes away a small part of our lives' meaning. How big is this loss? It depends.

Loss of a family member, like a parent, child, grandpa, or spouse can cause a great deal of grief. It can take years to recover fully. Sometimes, it takes years to recover completely because what is gone is irreplaceable.

This can also happen if we lose a loved pet or if we have a serious health problem. These are extremely difficult losses and can be very hard to overcome.

Other losses are more modest. What do I feel if an object is dear to me, something I received from a friend or something very useful? Naturally, I'm sad.

This happens when we lose something abstract. Back to the employment instance. My job made it feel valuable. I feel less valued now that I have lost my job. Their decisions will less reflect my views and take into account my needs. I feel scared, but also I feel sad. This sadness is due to my sense of loss in something abstract, such as value.

Sadness is like that, a testament to how important what we lost for us was.

It's hard to deal with sadness. First, let our brains process the events and plan for the changes in our lives that will result from this loss. The next step is to search for other resources that can be used to replace the resources lost. This will allow us to process the situation and help us find other resources that will meet our needs.

What is the purpose behind sadness?

It helps us to deal with loss. The sadness that we feel makes it easier to accept the loss. It's as though our brain had a few days to set aside all other activities to deal with the loss. Sadness helps our brain recognize the value of what was lost. It prevents us becoming indifferent.

Also, sadness encourages others to help us. The deeper the sadness, the more you cry. You will also notice changes in your voice and body language. All of these actions stimulate compassion and help to others. It's as though our brain is recruiting other brains to help with our loss processing by inducing these changes in our behavior.

Even the thought of losing someone we love or something can make us sad. This motivates us to give and receive more love and protection.

Sadness should be treated as any other emotion. It's the right response to grieve the loss of an important person or thing.

How does an autistic person handle emotions?

So far, we know that:

Happiness is when we are able to use a resource that fulfills a need. It doesn't matter if we need it or someone else's.

Fear arises when the brain predicts that a resource which meets our needs could be lost or damaged.

We feel anger when justice isn't being done.

Disgust can be caused by the loss of mental or bodily energy or when someone or something wears us down.

Unexpected stimuli are often met with surprise.

It is a sad thing to lose a resource. It's a means of coping.

Autism is characterized by difficulties in processing emotion-related information. This means that autistic people don't always understand how and why they are feeling certain emotions.

What is the practical application of this concept?

Take a look at the following examples to see the difference.

First, picture a young, neurotypical child losing his favorite toy. What happens next?

His brain registers his loss.

His brain tells his body to change in order to help him process the loss. These new sensations are called sadness.

It is often accompanied with a strong desire and need to get up in order to see his loved one. His brain sees other people as a potential source of support. His brain initiates the crying response because it knows that this will signal the distress of his brain to other brains, and recruit their assistance.

At the same moment, the child is afraid. How will life change after the favorite toy has gone? This causes his stomach to shrink and makes him more anxious.

His brain causes him to feel the need for sharing his fears with mother.

The young man is also feeling angry. "How could I be so stupid and loose my bear?" He says it aloud. This allows his mother the opportunity to hear what the boy is thinking. Her wisdom, comforting words and gestures can help him to cope with the loss.

Let's picture a young man living with autism in this exact situation.

His brain registers his loss.

Communication between areas processing loss and the rest the brain is inadequacies.

Although he feels upset, he doesn't feel any sadness or fear.

His body might feel ashamed of the thought of reaching for help. His psyche is often exhausted by social interaction. This is because he is dealing now with all these unpleasant sensations.

He is now calm and locked within himself. He feels angry, but isn't sure why. He also doesn't have the ability to express the distressing images or thoughts running through his mind.

His mother observes this behavior change and approaches him to find out why. The young man cannot explain the changes in his behavior.

He may try to cry, but depending on his autism level, he may end up making other sounds or yelling. He is unable to communicate well with his brain in this critical time because several parts of it aren't working together.

The inner turmoil he feels is so overwhelming that he finds it hard to sleep, and starts rocking back and forth in his chair.

His mother tries comfortingly to hug him but he resists. He sees physical contact as just one more thing in his overwhelmed brain.

The mother steps back. Her son was humming and flapping his arms, which made her feel dejected.

He starts to calm down gradually later.

We will soon know exactly what happened in steps 8, 9 and 10. We will soon know what happened in steps 8 and 9.

As you can see, forcing an autistic young boy to explain his problems can quickly be met with politeness. One might conclude that the young man with autism is rude and aggressive if they don't have any knowledge.

A wise person is able to see the bigger picture and can say, "Right Now." This young man struggles with distressing thoughts, strong feelings, and difficult emotions. These sensations cause his brain to be unable to process many of the feelings. I'll let him go for now, and then I'll try to get him involved at a later date."

The reader now belongs to the elite of those who are more able to understand things. Share your knowledge to help others.

You can have multiple emotions at once and in different degrees

Autism is not only difficult to understand emotions, which are often so abstract, but also the difficulty in feeling the emotion. Another difficulty associated with autism is the intensity of your emotional reactions.

Imagine your whole family agreeing to go to a museum this weekend. Saturday morning, the Asperger's child is eager to go on the trip. The family cannot make it due to an unexpected issue. Everyone is disappointed. However, the Asperger child reacts like the end of the world.

It appears as if there were only "black", "white", and no shades of grey. Either everything is fine or it's the end. There is no middle ground between 0 and 10, so it appears that the level or sadness, anger or fear are either at 0 or 10.

A person with autism can't understand what emotion he's feeling, except when it is already present at a very high level.

This can be caused either by problems in the region responsible for detecting contractions of your stomach, or by an inability of your stomach to associate contractions with an external stimulus.

It's almost like there's a plate full of spoiled food in front me. My brain isn't able to make the connection. I find it difficult to relate the disgust I feel to the spoiled food. I continue eating the rotten food because of this. Then, as I'm already nauseated I realize it was the food.

Why does it happen?

There are two possible causes: The responsible areas may not be functioning properly or the "cables" connecting them to the rest the brain are incorrectly connected. The message is not getting through. Until it's too late, the entire picture does not reach the conscious mind.

Neurotypical people can also do the reverse. He can calm his fears by letting go of them. However, autistic individuals have a lot more difficulty with this. While his conscious mind would like to relax, it seems this command information never gets sent to the right place.

Autism sufferers often have trouble controlling their temperament. Sometimes he explodes even though he doesn't want. We'll talk about this later.

However, for now, we are asking: How can this concrete understanding of emotion be applied in a way to benefit both autistic persons and their families? Let's see.

Practical emotional intelligence for the autistic

The concept of emotion intelligence is abstract. To make it more concrete, it will be divided into two main concepts:

The ability to identify and describe emotions, as well as the circumstances that trigger them. This involves being able to identify the emotions by name and understanding what situations usually trigger them.

Example: Understanding that an injustice causes anger can help you recognize that sadness can result from a loss.

Being able modulate or control emotions.

Example: Being capable of calming down when you are angry or scared, and being capable of comforting someone who is sad.

Next, we'll look at how to apply all that we've learned so far to each area.

Happiness: Identifying and dealing

How do you define happiness?

Happiness doesn't just mean laughing. Happiness is defined as a pleasant sensation that our bodies experience. If we experience this pleasant sensation, we can ask ourselves the following questions:

Did I meet my needs?

What did I do to contribute to the well-being of someone else?

Have I ever felt more self-confidence?

Did I receive any compliments?

Do I have a basic need for sleeping, eating, and rest?

Do you believe there will soon be something positive? What?

How does happiness affect you?

Happiness encourages us to share ideas and experience with others. We have a natural curiosity, a willingness to interact with others and explore the world around us -- even if our autism or social difficulties are present. Aspergers can be happy if they are able to talk about their favorite topic with another person. When happy, someone with a more profound form of autism may try to make contact with the outside. A person with autism may want to interact with the outside world because they are hungry.

What is the best thing to make someone happy?

We feel happy when we can do something to help another person. It fulfills our inherent need to be helpful to others.

We feel happy in the same way that we are fulfilled.

Furthermore, our expectations and belief in the fulfillment of our needs make us happy.

"Happiness" can also be understood as "satisfaction" or "hope".

The "negative emotions"

In the next pages, we'll be looking at the "negative" emotions. It's not that these emotions are necessarily negative, but rather that they are often associated with uncomfortable sensations that we don't enjoy feeling for long periods. These sensations can include tightness in the stomach, tingling sensations, muscle tension and changes to heart rhythm and breathing rate.

It's also difficult to recognize them because they share all of these characteristics. This is the problem. We need to see beyond sensations.

As such, we will be focusing on another aspect.

These emotions have a relationship with (1) our needs, and (2) the resources our brain believes are available to meet them.

In this sense, "resources" includes both people and things.

Do not be alarmed if you find it all too abstract. The next pages will give you many concrete examples to aid in understanding and clarity.

Help someone in fear by identifying them and providing support

Are you feeling unwell? How can you tell if they are being caused or fear? These are some questions to ask:

Do you think there is someone in your life I would flee to if it were possible?

Is there anyone or something that I can harm?

Is it possible that one of my resources or me is in danger?

Will there be anything that could potentially harm me in the near future?

Is it possible to meet someone who could hurt me or affect my resources?

Are there resources or anyone I am at risk of losing?

Am I at Risk of Not Being able to Access a Resource That Meets My Needs?

If we answer yes to any of these questions, then we most likely feel fear. Fear is not the only emotion you may feel. But, it's only one.

How to handle fear

If we cannot escape the things we feel are harmful, there are at least three options.

Change the odds. Believe that what you fear is unlikely to happen.

Have a plan B. Be positive that we are ready for anything, even if it's bad.

Summon allies in order to defeat the threat This means asking for help from other people. This means talking to others and telling them about the future. That's telling them our fears. These people can help us in many different ways. They can help us to create a plan A to handle any negative events that may occur. They can help us think better. These bad things are likely to happen? A friend would help us with options 2 and 1.

How can I help someone who is afraid?

These suggestions can also be used:

The same questions you asked above can be used to assist the person in identifying the cause of his fear.

Take on the role of an ally for him or her:

You can help the person to re-evaluate their chances of something bad happening.

He or she can be helped to develop a plan B. The strategy that increases confidence in the person's ability to deal effectively with any situation, whether it is a nightmare or its aftermath.

Help this person to find more friends.

The threat to someone experiencing fear will look smaller if more people are available to assist.

Remember that fear is like all other emotions and exists in degrees. This means that we can reduce the fear level even if it is impossible to eliminate. We can help them brainstorm ways to lessen the threat.

Calming someone mad by identifying and soothing them

Are your unpleasant feelings a sign of anger or frustration? They could be. These questions might be helpful:

Has there been anything I consider inhumane?

Is there anything that I feel is unfair?

Is there something I don't like about someone?

Is anyone or anything preventing me fulfilling my needs?

Are there any rules I believe to have been violated?

Is there an urgent need of mine which isn't being met or that I need urgently?

Is there anything that I feel has been crossed by another?

Is there something in my life that I should try to change?

Answering yes to any of these question is a sign that anger triggers the negative emotions you are experiencing.

How to deal avec anger

An injustice is something that makes us angry. Furthermore, our brain tends to be focused on resources and need, so to manage anger, you must identify the injustice and then relate it to our resources. When anger gives rise to another emotion, we know we are successful in our detective work. This emotion is more closely related to the problem.

Do you find this too complex? Let's examine some examples.

If I am annoyed by someone who horns at or tries to ram me in the road, I might ask: "What are my needs?" It might be that I have a need for peace of thought or to see people treat one another well. Once I recognize these needs, I stop viewing the other person's threat as something I must eliminate as quickly as possible. Why? Because my focus has shifted.

I remember thinking before:

"Who thinks he is?"

"What? "What?

"I have it when people hunk at me."

"Why aren't you honking?" Can't you see that you're the one who almost struck me?

All of these thoughts were ripples resulting from the lightning fast evaluation my unconscious made on the situation.

That one act, "someone shouting at me, even though I had done nothing wrong," was enough to make me feel unjustified.

All of these mental processing, evaluations, and mental processing occurred without my conscious attention. Furthermore, my brain activated stress, which transformed my entire body into war machines. It caused my conscious mind to be filled with disturbing thoughts about the other individual. After that, my conscious mind took control of the situation.

Do you know how the world has changed? I was at peace a few seconds ago. Then, someone honked. Now, I'm a new man.

All of these stressors are affecting my breathing patterns as well as my heart beat. My head is filled of enemy images. I'm feeling angry.

Fortunately, I knew the right thing to do. I kept asking my self:

"Why is my brain focusing on this situation so much?" Why does my brain consider'someone honking to me' a matter for life and death? What are the important needs here?

As my focus shifted, my underlying rage also changed. Anger eventually gave way to curiosity. To be my own detective, curiosity drove me. I never stopped looking for the causes of my anger.

Inquiring questions causes my unconscious mind and body to be preoccupied with finding the answers. Then, I realize how much the whole situation has affected me and my peace of mind. Either I'm sad or afraid, depending on how the situation plays out.

Once the needs have been identified I am empowered and able to make the best decisions. I can ask myself "How can I protect my needs?"

149

Then, other thoughts will arise in my head. Maybe you'll find answers like these:

I can reach out and touch him. Perhaps then he'll stop honking. I'll be able to regain my peace and mind.

I'll wait until traffic moves again. If that doesn't happen, excuse me once more and then drive away.

I can distract and cause me to think about other things.

I can count to 10 and take deep breaths.

I can picture the consequences of my anger. How would it affect my reputation My family? The family members of the man honking?

What would make me happy in 20 years? Recalling how cool I was under fire or how violently I reacted to provocations.

Was anger helpful?

Yes. Anger showed me how my world had changed. But, anger wasn't helpful for me in dealing with the problem.

Sometimes, turning anger into an emotion can be hard. What happens when my son is brought home with a bruised face, and I find out that he was beaten up by two bullies? I'm enraged. That's normal. That was no accident.

This anger can be very useful. If I do unto them as they have done to me, the violence will only escalate. And the consequences will get worse than a bruised nose. It is possible that people will die. However, I can't simply stand by and let it happen. My anger is too intense to allow me to stay still. Anger is helpful in this situation. How do we deal with it?

First, I must determine the needs. These include: (1) the well-being of my child, (2) the safety and security of my child at school, (3) justice, and so forth.

I then ask myself "How can we meet those needs?"

These two steps allow me to shift my focus. Instead of thinking "how can they make me pay?" I think "How can you meet your needs?"

This helps me come up with solutions.

Report a problem to the school authorities.

Get legal advice about what you should do next.

Consider changing schools.

My child should carefully analyze his school habits in order to find ways to make changes that will prevent future confrontations.

Talk to your bullies' parents.

It is worth talking to bullies in the presence a school authority as well as the bullies' parents.

Enroll your child in a program which provides guidance and support on dealing with these problems.

Consider seeking professional help for parents and children in such situations.

You can remind yourself that bullies have been dealt with successfully by many people before you, without resorting to violence.

Ask for help from mature adults who have suffered bullying, and who were able solve the problem peacefully.

Find books and articles online about the subject.

So, anger can be used to its full potential. It alerted me about injustices and stopped me from overlooking them. I was motivated by anger to act. Because of the threat hovering above my boy, it might have even turned into fear. It isn't paralyzing fear. Instead, it is the fear based in facts that drives me to take actions to help my children avoid the outcome they fear.

This is why anger is useful: it helps us identify the causes and resources of our anger. Why? Because it allowed us to witness injustice without being forced to move.

How can you help someone who is angry?

It is possible to empathize and understand the importance of justice.

What if anger is directed against you?

If someone is being aggressive or bullying you, it takes a lot more emotional intelligence to deal with the situation. Many bullying victims are not able to handle this type of psychological violence.

Bullying often starts in pre-school, continues at the workplace and spreads through other social interactions.

Even if someone diagnosed with autism is able process emotions to the point where they can help others feeling angry, it's much more difficult for him to defend himself against bullying.

Because bullying requires a prompt and appropriate response. The autistic person can't just sit at home and think about how to protect himself. He must either use his smartphone to learn how to react or he will not be able to.

It is therefore essential to be able to access simple and straightforward techniques.

The best way to deal with an aggressive person is Dr. David M. Burns's adjunct professor emeritus within the Department of Psychiatry and Behavioral Sciences of Stanford University School of Medicine.

I'm referring to the technique of disarming. This technique is simple to master and very easy for you to use. It will not work all the times, especially if someone is trying to make problems. When we are dealing with criticism or accusations, however, it can be quite useful.

Simply put, when someone calls or accuses you of something, there are two options to disarm them.

Calm the person and find a way of agreeing with him. Try to find truth in the comments, regardless of whether they are right or wrong. This takes out criticism.

Ask for details. Ask questions that will help you learn more about him and what he doesn't like about you. This helps to foster a healthy dialog.

If someone is aggressive to you, it only makes things worse. Only aggressiveness can work if we make the other person fearful of us. This mentality however only leads to increased violence, more hospitalizations, and more deaths.

Conversely, if someone is being critical or aggressive towards you, finding a way of agreeing with them can help calm them down. It is also a good way to start a dialogue towards peace by asking for examples. If the person is aggressive, it's not surprising that he will apologize.

The key to the technique's success is that lying is prohibited. The only way to agree with the other person is if he's right.

What if they're wrong? There are two possible ways to get around it

Accept that sometimes you do what you are accused of.

You agree that the person in question has the right to be mad at that situation.

How does it work in practice? Let's examine some examples.

Example 1

Aggressive phrase: Your worthlessness!

Disarming answer 1 : Yes, I do make mistakes (agreeing avec the aggressor). Do you think of any specifics? (Asking for details).

Answer 2 to the Disarming Question: I understand that your emotions are upset by what happened. (Asking for details).

Example 2

Adverse phrase: Why don't you ever do something right?

Disarming Answer 1: I see you did something differently (agreeing). Can you tell me? (Asking for details)

Disarming Answer 2: I see, you like things done right (agreeing). Please tell me about the mistakes I made. (Asking for details).

Answer 3: Disarming. I can understand. It's frustrating when people don't want to help (agreeing it is normal for such situations to be disturbing to a person). Could you tell where I could have been more useful? (Asking for details).

Example 3

Aggressive phrase

Disarming Answer 1: Sometimes I don't get it. (agreeing). Could you please explain to me the things you think I should understand better? (Ask for details, but recognize that even if you think you know something, there is always more to learn.

Disarming Answer 2: It must be frustrating for you when you want me learn something and I see that it isn't possible (agreeing). Out of all the things that you tried to teach me, which one are your thoughts about? (Asking for details).

If the accusation proves false, you can disarm the answer 3. (Asking for specifics, giving the person an opportunity of revealing what he is thinking).

Example 4

Aggressive phrase.

Disarming answer 1 : This is a possibility. I, too, don't like it. (Agreeing with most of the principles but not agreeing completely with the aggressive person's predictions). Can you tell me what areas I could improve upon? (Asking for information in a nonthreatening way).

Disarming Answer 2: This is really worrying you (agreeing that someone is concerned). Can you tell me why? (Asking for details).

In each instance, the aggressive sentence was used by someone in battle mode. Words were transformed into arrows by his mouth to try and pierce you.

Your non-contradictory responses send a clear message through the limbic system to the other person.

You are not considered a threat

This makes it easier to develop a pleasant dialog.

Aside from the disarming technique there is also a more effective method called "The Benjamin Franklin Effect".

The Benjamin Franklin effect

Benjamin Franklin was one among the founding fathers the United States. He is also recognized as the inventor the lightning rod.

In his autobiography he describes how and why he faced political opposition.

I heard from him that he had a book that was very rare and intriguing. I wrote him a letter expressing my desire to read it, and asking him to lend me the book for a few weeks. I sent it back in about a week and he said it instantly. The next time we met in the House [of Representatives], I heard him speak to me, something he had never done before. I returned it within a week with another note, expressing my gratitude for the favor. We became great friends and continued our friendship until his death. >>[3]

What makes a small favor so successful? Our brain is a congruent being, it turns out. It's as though our unconscious part of the brain said, "I don't really like that person, but... I did him an favor." It's hard to believe that I could have done him favors if he didn't love me. He must be a part of my life. This is more sensible than believing that I don't enjoy him.

This is what psychologists call the brain's need solve cognitive dissonances.

This is why people tend to love a product more when they have purchased it. It is almost like our subconscious brain is saying, "Well, although I was unsure if this product would be good or bad, I did purchase it." This surely means that I wasn't so uncertain as I thought.

All of this is understandable. It is possible that there is another reason.

One example is how people react when you ask for directions. Try it. Ask for directions next time your are on the street. You will be amazed at how people react to your questions.

What's happening?

As we all know, contributing to others' well-being is one of our most fundamental human needs. While someone may not notice it, being critical or aggressive can make you feel fulfilled if you do something that benefits another person.

Keep these things in mind. It can be a problem if a favor takes too much physical or mental energy.

If you can offer small favors, it may bring you a sense of satisfaction. The aggressive person has now associated "feeling good", with "doing well to you."

How can these principles be applied to win the respect of someone aggressive?

Ask for little favors. Simple things. Then, thank them for their kindness and gratitude. Yes, it might be hard to know exactly where to start. Here are some examples that will help you get started:

Can you please tell us what time it is? Thank you.

Where is our next class? We are so grateful for your kind words.

I would appreciate it if you could pass this on to me. Thank you. It is a great feeling.

This is so nice. That was so kind. We are grateful.

Ask for advice or opinions.

Hi! I know you are a great gamer of [name the game]. Please help me to beat this level.

I'm confused between these two options. Can I have your help?

You should always ask for something you feel satisfied doing. It doesn't have to be complicated.

Some bullies in school are resilient, but persistence in being kind will bring about positive results.

Help someone who is experiencing disgust by helping them identify it.

What questions can you ask to determine if the unsightly sensations you feel are a sign of disinterest?

Do I feel nauseous?

Do I feel like vomiting?

Is it possible that I will do something that I didn't want?

Will I meet someone who wastes my mental energies?

Do I have a relationship with someone who is wasting my mental or bodily energy?

Was it necessary to stop doing something I liked?

Is there anything in your life that you wish wasn't?

Are you feeling mentally tired or depressed?

Is my brain refusing to accept everything? Even thinking.

Disgust is often difficult to identify and goes unnoticed. It is difficult to recognize and often goes unnoticed.

How do you deal with the disgust?

It is best to treat disgust in two ways. It is essential to rest your mind when you are tired. You should be calm and lying down.

But, sometimes physical rest does not necessarily mean your mind will recover. Why?

Now imagine you feel nauseated or disgusted at the thought of dealing with a troublesome person tomorrow. Because your mind will be focused on the subject, it won't help to stay still. This can cause you to lose your mental stamina. This may mean that it is necessary to take part in activities you truly enjoy. This can be a difficult task for autistic people.

Tony Attwood who is considered to be the world's top Asperger's expert, says that for every hour spent with people, someone diagnosed should spend an extra hour alone, resting their mind. We'll be discussing the impact that people have on autism later in this book.

Just for the moment, remember that anger is a strong emotion which draws us closer towards the situation and makes us want to take action. Disgust, on the other hand, leads us away from the situation and motivates our actions.

We can also try to determine what resources and needs are involved, or underlying disgust. Most of the time, the need to rest is what you feel. However, if you find that getting away and resting doesn't alleviate your disgust, it could be a sign of other needs.

How can I help someone who is suffering from disgust?

It is crucial to help the person move away from the stimulus which caused the reaction. This is not the right way to make the person continue to process the stimulus. It's also not the best idea to keep them in contact with the person who is triggering their disgust. Why? It can lead to disgust that is so strong it causes people to become irritable. Forcing an autistic person into interacting when he is tired can lead to a nervous breakdown and a meltdown.

Helping someone surprise you

Surprise typically lasts for a few minutes. If the surprise lasts more than a few minutes, we call it shock. We often use this term to refer to our shock and state that we are still processing or assimilating what happened.

These are some questions that can help us determine if we should be surprised by the unpleasant sensations we feel.

What was it that I didn't expect?

Have you ever witnessed something shocking?

Have you ever experienced something that has confused you?

How to manage surprise?

It is essential to take time to understand everything. You can also benefit from the support of an understanding friend with autism.

How do I help someone who is confused or feeling shocked?

Surprise can signal that you need to learn new and unanticipated information. This can be done with some well-placed queries. These include:

What happened?

Why was this surprising to you?

What were your expectations?

Why do you think things went differently?

How do you see the future of things because of what happened?

What are the negative side effects of what has happened?

What are some of the good points?

How can you cope with the negative side effects?

Who can you help?

What can I do to help you now?

We want the person to create a narrative. These questions will be answered by the narrative.

Why did this happen?

How did it make things better?

What can I do now to adjust to the events that have occurred?

The person will understand this and be able overcome shock. The story isn't over. Depending on what you now know about the future, it is possible to feel scared, disgusted and angry.

Helping someone in distress.

Are you feeling sad? Ask yourself these questions.

Was it someone or a pet that I have lost?

Is someone you love or your pet sick?

Have I lost anyone I loved?

Are you in love with someone?

Is there someone I wish I could have with me, but who isn't?

What happened that I lost my self-respect? Or my desire to live my life?

What health problems have I been diagnosed with?

Do I believe that bad things are coming to someone I love or to something else?

All these questions all share the same theme: loss. It doesn't really matter what the loss is, it can be real or imaginary.

How to handle sadness and be a helper?

At least two goals can be achieved to make sadness less.

We allow our mind to think in a way that is most comfortable for us.

Sometimes, it can take quite a while to get through a big loss like the death, or the inability to bury a loved one.

We find a way to use the resources or strategies that are available to us in order meet our needs.

Two types of questions can be asked to speed up the pursuit of these two goals.

These questions are meant to be answered by others and help them understand why they lost it.

These are questions that can be used to help establish a link between the resource being lost and his needs.

Asking questions helps them to think about how to make changes in their lives to increase their ability to meet their needs.

These questions are helpful in helping the person to determine how other resources can be used for their same needs.

Let's see some examples. These questions should not be asked unless the person is ready. Depending upon the extent of the loss, you might need to wait several weeks or even days before the person is able to make a decision about what happened.

These questions are meant to be answered by others and help them understand why they lost it.

Why did you love this person?

What do you like most about his personality and how did it make you feel?

How did this person help?

What did you do?

Which ways do you think you rely on him?

How did your life change after the death of this person?

Why did your pet like you?

What did you do together?

What are your biggest regrets?

How has your world changed since then?

Why was this object so significant to you

What were you using it for?

How has your life changed after you have lost it all?

Someone who loses a brother may have experienced more than one loss. He has lost a friend. Sometimes, it may be necessary for several people to assume each of these roles.

It's about not trying to replace the deceased person. It's simply that, even after such a tragic loss, you still need to have friends, confidants, playmates.

Our chances of coping with a loss are higher if we find new ways to help. However, no one can replace the loss, but there may be many people willing to try to satisfy the same needs or even more. This will decrease the sense of despair.

The following questions will help someone locate new resources that meet his needs:

How many other valued people do you know?

What kind help do they need to succeed?

What can we do to help them today?

What can you do to help others fulfill your desire to contribute to their wellbeing?

How can these people help you?

What would be your dream pet animal?

Why?

Think about the day when you'll be able to care and take care of another pet.

What do you think of going to your friend's house to play and his pet?

What other objects do you have that can help you achieve the same goal of the lost object,

You could ask, "What other objects have you got that can help you remember this person?"

Reverse Engineering Emotions

This chapter provides a concrete understanding on emotions and their role within our lives. This concrete understanding allows you to reverse engineer emotions. How?

The questions discussed earlier in this chapter can be used by an autistic person to discover the injustice that his brain has detected.

These questions assist the autistic person in performing manual tasks that his brain should have done automatically. This is a good thing because the neuroplastic qualities of our brain will allow us to automate this manual process over time.

The person with autism can learn more and process things quicker by training. You may find 2 or 3 most frequent needs after repeating this process several times.

"I suffered injustice!" This means that my need to be treated with respect was not considered. This makes me mad. It makes me feel angry, but it also makes me sad if people lose respect for my work. What can I do?

This is a huge improvement over what used to take many hours or minutes.

All of this assumes the person with autism has an atypical form of the condition such as Asperger's syndrome.

If someone has a deeper form autism, in which communication skills are affected, it may be harder for them to understand these abstract concepts. He might need to do this for many years. For people with autism spectrum disorders, however, it may take him many years to read this chapter. This chapter may change their approach to the strange sensations they experience in their body and affect how they feel about emotions. This understanding can be life-changing.

Staying on the topic, you might have noticed autistic individuals who wiggle their hands, rock on a stool, or make noises using their mouths. What causes these behaviors? How should parents interpret these behaviors. We'll explore this topic in the next section.

Chapter 10: How to Uncover the Mysteries of Stimming

Imagine talking to someone about a favorite topic. You are passionate, but you keep noticing how the other person taps their foot. You don't notice this. You argue, "I am almost done with this explanation." You will find more amazing ideas the more you explain.

Your attention is not even on the next minute. Only your voice is heard. The other person isn't looking at you any more, he just stares at the watch wondering when the conversation will stop. His hands are not still. He crosses his arms and then moves his hand to his hips.

You are impatient, it's obvious. We are curious to know why people become impatient.

At least two reasons can be given for this. It is polite to show the other person you are done with the conversation. These movements can also be used to calm us.

It's well known that movement can calm you down. The more you do, the better. Multiple clinical studies confirm the antidepressant and calming effects of regular exercise. Everyone who has ever been home after a hard day at work and felt exhausted can relate to the desire to relax and get to sleep.

Parents also notice this in their children. They feel calmer when they spend time outside, running, and playing with the ball.

You might like to try it. If you're feeling anxious, go for a stroll. Walking will help calm you down.

Let's remember this basic characteristic of autism. The brain areas responsible for modeling emotions doesn't work properly when someone with autism is present. This in practice means that the autistic person will have difficulty controlling their feelings.

We have seen the effects of this on the way an autistic child handles his emotions, compared with a neurotypical boy.

Intuitively, a young neurotypical feels the need to vent. To distract himself from an activity or think about other options.

Young autists use a different approach to decrease the intensity of their emotions. He flaps his arms, jumps, dances in a chair, moves erratically and pulls his hair.

Any action that reduces the intensity and difficulty of his emotions can help him to understand them better.

These movements are known in English as "stimming".

Some stimming may not be so good. Some strategies of stimming may be harmful, such as hurting oneself or another person, overthrowing other things, acting violently, or shouting at others. What should we do?

While you need to stop your child hurting themselves or others, how can this be done in a way that your child is able to relax?

How to handle the stimming caused by moderate autism (such as Asperger's)?

Being a parent can be difficult watching your child flailing his hands. It's okay to feel the need for your child to stop. However, it would be a horrible thing to do. Why?

Because stimming can be used by autistic people to control their nervous tension, and increase the intensity of their emotions. Everyone has the need to control unpleasant sensations in their bodies. The strategy of choice for autistic patients is stimming.

To stop stimming the autistic person develops nervous tics, such as tremors on the lips or eyelids. This can lead to nervous breakdowns. It is almost certain that an autistic person will fall into depression if stimming is prohibited.

It might seem hard to hear. However, there isn't much one can do. Just as breathing is part of being human, so too is stimming.

What can you do if your children are exhibiting destructive behavior like stimming?

It's important to encourage children to try a more harmless way of stimming. Teach your child how stim. Your child may think you're crazy if you tell other parents about the benefits to rolling in bed and flapping his hands.

It's your son.

His brain lacks the neurochemical connections required to regulate the intensity and frequency of his emotions. You can't teach your son how to properly stim. It's only a matter time before destructive stimming causes trouble and brings pain to your entire family.

Teaching your child how to stim should begin as soon and as quickly as possible. If he experiences unpleasant sensations, such as wanting to run away or scream at someone, it is important to take him to the nearest public bathroom or another designated place. He can then flap his hands or jump until calm.

Once he can understand the concept, use concrete teaching techniques to explain emotions to him. Use as many examples of his emotions as possible. Your points can be illustrated with pictures, videos, or drawings. These examples can be modified to fit the autism level of an adult, a child, or teenager.

If possible, include examples that are related to his hobbies. This theme can be used as a basis for examples if he is passionate about trains. If your child is passionate about Star Wars, use that. Do this, and your child will be forever changed.

Your child will be able to understand the unpleasant sensations and help you find better ways for him to calm down. These can include sitting alone in a quiet area while your child engages in a favorite hobby, such as art or listening to music.